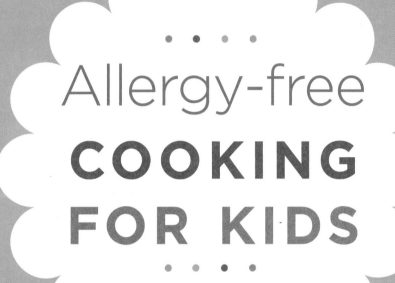

Allergy-free
COOKING
FOR KIDS

More than **90** Yummy
Savories & Sweets

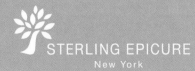

STERLING EPICURE
New York

contents

Children with food allergies can really feel left out, especially at parties: "If everyone else can eat birthday cake, then why can't I?" And it's hard on parents—you worry your child may eat something they will severely react to, but it's heartbreaking having to tell them they're not allowed the same food as everyone else.

Why my child?

Good question, but unfortunately there is no easy answer. We do know that genetics has something to do with it, with the children of allergy sufferers more likely to have allergies themselves. There is a 50–70 percent chance that children will develop allergies if both parents are allergy sufferers. The risk diminishes if only one parent has an allergy, but is still higher than if neither parent has ever had an allergy. According to the Center for Disease Control, 4 percent of children in the US under the age of 18 have food allergies. Eight foods account for the vast majority of all food-allergy reactions. They are cow's milk, eggs, peanuts, tree-nuts, fish, shellfish, soy beans, and wheat.

What's the difference?

A food allergy is not the same as food intolerance. Food allergies are abnormal immune system responses to something we eat. The immune system incorrectly thinks that a certain food is a danger to the body and releases harmful chemicals into the bloodstream.

Food intolerances are adverse reactions to certain foods, but do not involve the immune system. With intolerances you can generally eat a little of the offending food before experiencing any symptoms. Symptoms normally include tummy and bowel upsets, bloating, hives, and headaches.

Food allergies are generally more serious than food intolerances, as they can be life-threatening.

Common offenders

The foods most commonly associated with allergic reactions are gluten, milk, eggs, peanuts, tree nuts, and shellfish. Luckily, there are many alternatives and substitutes available that you can use in place of these offenders, often without your child even realizing.

Nuts are especially tricky as nut meal is used in many cakes and cookies, making it impossible to detect if you don't know the source. They are also commonly found in chocolates, nougat, cereals, and stir-fries. Always check the label of store-bought food for traces of nuts.

Gluten can lurk in processed foods, especially in foods like seafood or meat substitutes, processed meats, candies, soups, gravies, and sauces.

If you have an egg allergy watch out for baked goods, ice creams, custards, soups, fresh pasta, and many desserts like soufflés and crème caramel.

So what should you do?

It's possible, and very important, to make delicious food that not only your child will like, but that the whole family and your children's friends will like as well. That way they won't feel left out or like they're different from everyone else. The recipes here are for delicious gluten-free, dairy-free, and egg-free food that will be quickly gobbled up by everyone. They cover every mealtime, snack time, and even party time and, best of all, none of it looks in the least like "special" food.

While many of the larger supermarkets are increasing the number of gluten-, nut-, dairy-, and egg-free, etc., products on their shelves, your local health food store is always a good place to source those harder-to-find items. They are also usually more than happy to order any special requests. Also, check out web sites specializing in allergy-free products.

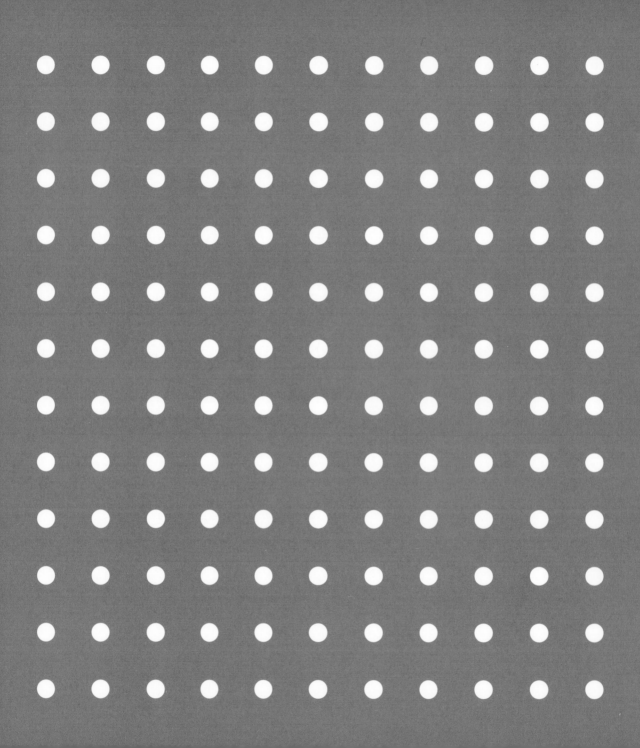

gluten-free

A gluten allergy doesn't sentence you to a life of boring food—as these fabulous recipes show.

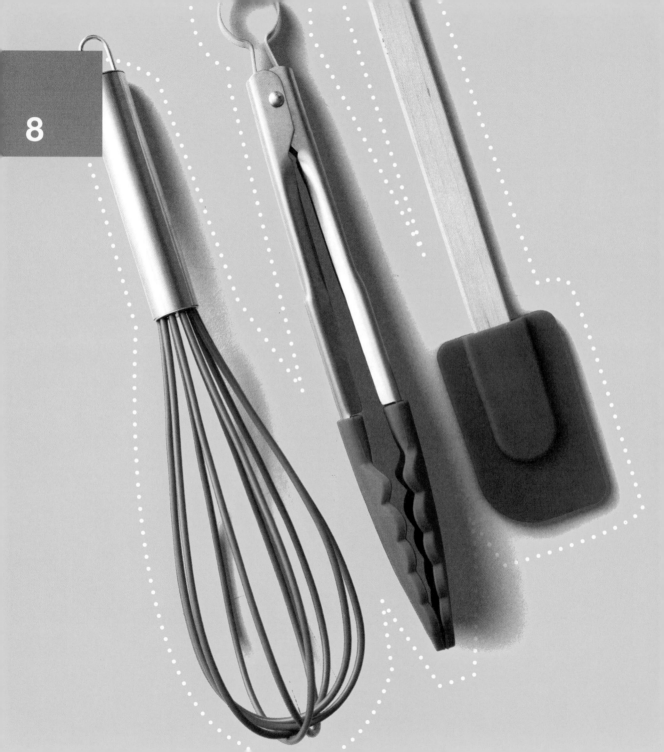

My favorite recipes

....
....
....
....
....
....
....
....
....

Breakfast Pancakes, eggs, granola—these gluten-free dishes taste so good the whole family will happily devour them.

banana pancakes

This recipe is also nut-free.

1¼ cups gluten-free
   self-rising flour
¼ cup brown rice flour
2 tablespoons superfine sugar
1 cup milk
3 eggs
3 tablespoons butter, melted
2 large bananas (1 lb), thickly sliced
¼ cup brown sugar

1 Sift flours and sugar into medium bowl. Whisk milk, eggs, and half the butter in medium pitcher. Gradually whisk milk mixture into flour mixture until smooth.
2 Heat large heavy-based frying pan over medium heat; brush with a little of the remaining butter. Pour 2 tablespoons batter for each pancake into heated pan. Cook pancakes until bubbles appear on the surface; top pancakes with banana, sprinkle each pancake with a rounded teaspoon of brown sugar.
3 Flip pancakes over; cook until sugar has caramelized and banana is browned lightly. Cover to keep warm.
4 Repeat process to make a total of 12 pancakes, wiping out pan between each batch.

prep + cook time 25 minutes makes 12 nutritional count per pancake 179 calories; 5.1 g total fat (2.8 g saturated fat); 29.3 g carbohydrate; 0.9 g fiber; 3.3 g protein

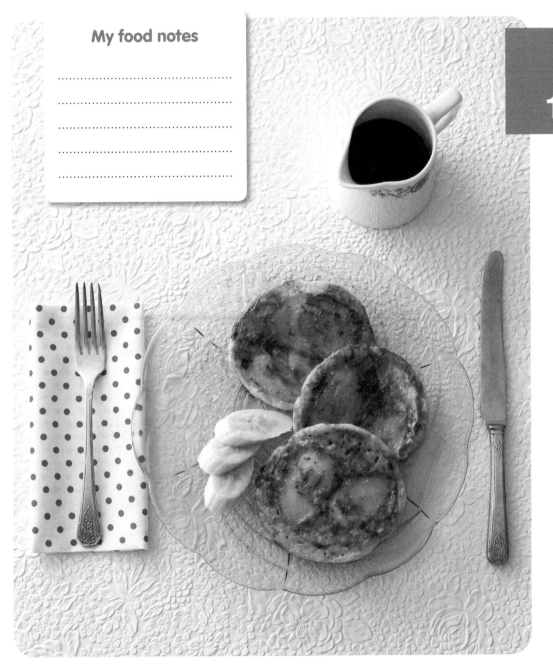

My food notes

....
....
....
....
....

Did you know? Banana plants are actually giant herbs. They're a great energy food and a good source of vitamin C and potassium. Cut bananas just before using as they discolor quickly.

Allergy-free cooking for kids gluten-free Breakfast

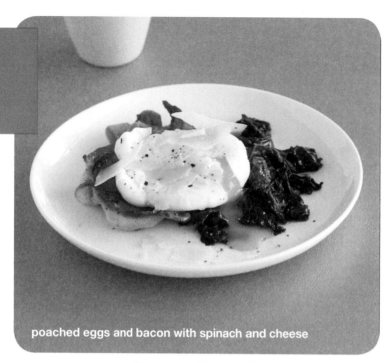

poached eggs and bacon with spinach and cheese

prep + cook time
15 minutes
serves 4
nutritional count
per serving
198 calories;
16.6 g total fat
(3.9 g saturated fat);
0.9 g carbohydrate;
2.1 g fiber;
23.6 g protein

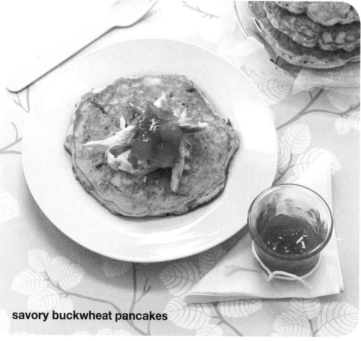

savory buckwheat pancakes

prep + cook time
30 minutes
makes 10
nutritional count
per pancake
332 calories;
8.1 g total fat
(2 g saturated fat);
38.2 g carbohydrate;
5.4 g fiber;
23.5 g protein

poached eggs and bacon with spinach and cheese

This recipe is also nut-free.

21 oz spinach, trimmed, coarsely chopped
4 gluten-free bacon strips (9 oz)
4 eggs
⅓ cup (1 oz) flaked pecorino cheese

1 Boil, steam, or microwave spinach until just wilted; drain. Cover to keep warm.
2 Heat large frying pan over medium heat; cook bacon until crisp. Drain on paper towels; cover to keep warm.
3 Half-fill the same pan with water; bring to the boil. Break one egg into small cup; slide into pan. Repeat with remaining eggs; when all eggs are in pan, allow water to return to the boil. Cover pan, turn off heat; stand about 4 minutes or until a light film of egg white sets over yolks. Using a slotted spoon, remove eggs, one at a time, from pan; place on paper towel-lined saucer to blot up poaching liquid.
4 Divide spinach among serving plates; top with bacon, egg, then cheese.

Use flaked parmesan cheese if pecorino is not available.

savory buckwheat pancakes

This recipe is also nut-free.

1 cup buckwheat flour
½ cup gluten-free all-purpose flour
3 teaspoons gluten-free baking powder
2 eggs
2 cups buttermilk
3 tablespoons butter, melted
1 medium zucchini (4 oz), coarsely grated
1 small carrot (2 oz), coarsely grated
½ cup (3 oz) fresh or frozen corn kernels

1 Sift flours and baking powder into large bowl; gradually whisk in eggs and buttermilk until smooth. Stir in butter and vegetables.
2 Spray a small frying pan over medium heat with cooking spray, pour ⅓ cup of the batter into pan; cook until bubbles appear on surface. Turn pancake; cook until browned lightly. Repeat with remaining batter to make a total of 10 pancakes.

Serve pancakes topped with shredded barbecued chicken and gluten-free mango chutney, if you like.

corn, cheese, and carrot omelettes

This recipe is also nut-free.

8 eggs
11 oz can creamed corn
1 large carrot (6 oz), coarsely grated
¼ cup finely chopped fresh
**   flat-leaf parsley**
½ cup (2 oz) coarsely grated reduced-fat
**   cheddar cheese**

1 Whisk eggs in medium bowl until combined; stir in remaining ingredients.
2 Spray a small frying pan with cooking spray and warm over medium heat; pour a quarter of the egg mixture into pan and cook until omelette is set. Fold omelette in half, slide onto plate; cover to keep warm.
3 Repeat process with remaining egg mixture to make three more omelettes.

prep + cook time 30 minutes **makes** 4 **nutritional count per serving** 278 calories; 14.7 g total fat (5.6 g saturated fat); 15.3 g carbohydrate; 4 g fiber; 19.6 g protein

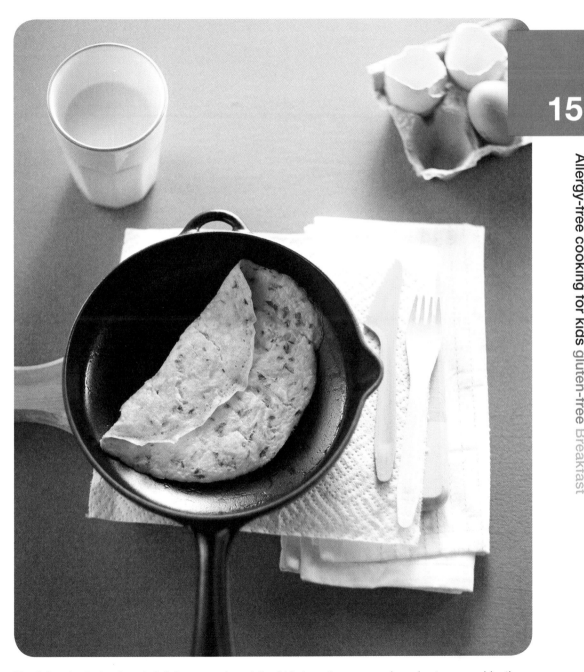

Healthy tip A simple yet delicious way to get the kids to eat more veggies: also try a combination of other vegetables such as zucchini, peppers, bean sprouts, scallions, spinach, and mushrooms.

16

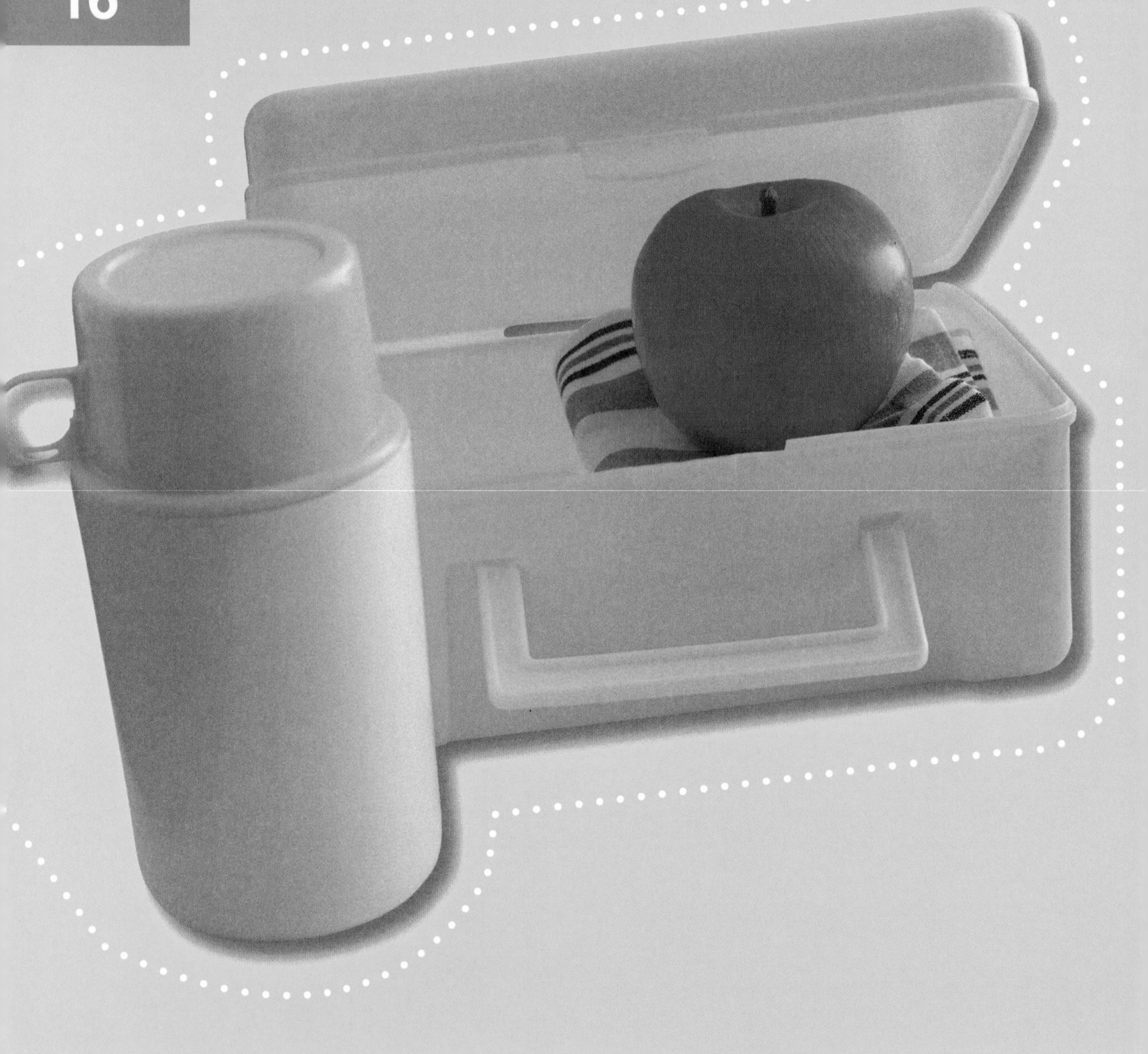

My favorite recipes

....

....

....

....

....

....

....

....

....

Always pack lunches with a frozen drink or an ice pack to keep them cool and fresh until lunchtime.

pizza pinwheels

This recipe is also nut-free.

1 stick butter, softened
1 tablespoon confectioners' sugar, sifted
2 egg yolks
1 cup (8 oz) cooked mashed potato, sieved
1 cup potato flour
½ cup brown rice flour
1 tablespoon gluten-free baking powder
⅓ cup tomato paste
about ¼ lb gluten-free thinly sliced ham,
    finely chopped
1 oz (about 1½ cups) baby spinach leaves
1½ cups (5 oz) pizza cheese

Pack pinwheels, wrapped in parchment, in lunchbox. Pinwheels can be stored in an airtight container in the refrigerator overnight, or frozen for up to 3 months.

1 Preheat oven to 425°F/400°F convection. Oil 7 x 11-inch baking pan.
2 Beat butter, confectioners' sugar, and yolks in small bowl with electric mixer until light and fluffy. Transfer mixture to large bowl; stir in mashed potato.
3 Add sifted dry ingredients; stir to make a soft dough. Knead dough lightly on floured surface until smooth. Roll dough between sheets of parchment to 8 x 12-inch rectangle.
4 Spread tomato paste over dough; sprinkle ham, spinach, and 1 cup of the cheese over the top.
5 Starting from long side, roll dough firmly using paper as a guide; trim ends. Cut roll into 12 slices; place pinwheels, cut-side up, in single layer, in pan. Bake 20 minutes. Remove pinwheels from oven, sprinkle remaining cheese over; bake 10 minutes more.

prep + cook time 50 minutes makes 12 nutritional count per pinwheel 230 calories; 13.4 g total fat (8 g saturated fat); 19.7 g carbohydrate; 1.1 g fiber; 7.4 g protein

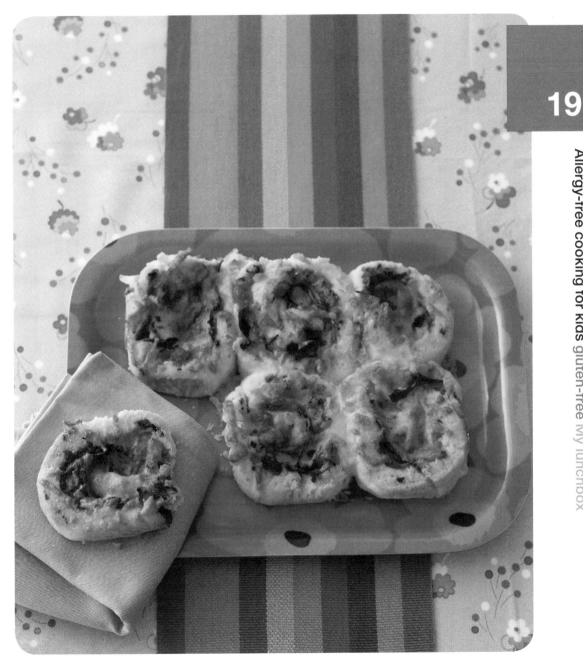

Helpful hint Pizza cheese is a commercial blend of processed grated mozzarella, parmesan, and cheddar cheeses. Use plain cheddar cheese if you like, or use a tasty or mature cheddar for extra bite.

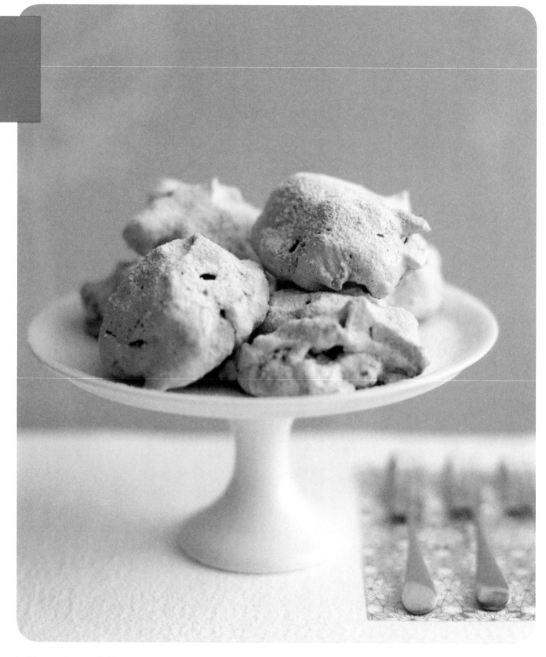

Did you know? The almond is closely related to the plum, apricot, and cherry. Almonds make a great snack as they contain more calcium than other nuts, and are rich in vitamins B and E, and iron.

cranberry chewies

This recipe is also dairy-free.

¾ cup (2 oz) sliced almonds
3 egg whites
½ cup superfine sugar
1 tablespoon (100% corn) cornstarch
1 teaspoon finely grated orange rind
¾ cup (4 oz) dried cranberries
1 tablespoon confectioners' sugar

1 Preheat oven to 325°F/300°F convection. Grease baking sheets; line with parchment.
2 Dry roast nuts in medium frying pan over medium-low heat until browned lightly; remove from pan.
3 Beat egg whites in small bowl with electric mixer until soft peaks form. Gradually add sugar, beating until sugar dissolves; transfer to medium bowl. Fold in sifted cornstarch, rind, cranberries, and nuts, in two batches.
4 Drop heaped tablespoons of mixture about 1½ inch apart onto baking sheets; bake about 30 minutes. Stand on sheets 5 minutes before transferring to wire rack to cool. Dust with sifted confectioners' sugar to serve.

prep + cook time 50 minutes makes 18 nutritional count per chewie 71 calories; 1.9 g total fat (0.1 g saturated fat); 12 g carbohydrate; 0.5 g fiber; 1.3 g protein

omelette wrap

This recipe is also nut-free.

cooking oil spray
4 eggs, beaten lightly
2 tablespoons gluten-free mayonnaise
2 teaspoons finely chopped fresh dill
1 teaspoon lemon juice
3½ oz watercress, trimmed
3½ oz smoked salmon
½ Lebanese cucumber (2 oz),
    seeded, cut into matchsticks

1 Spray medium frying pan with cooking oil; cook half the eggs over medium heat, swirling pan to make a thin omelette. Remove from pan; cool on parchment-covered wire rack. Repeat with remaining eggs.
2 Combine mayonnaise, dill, and juice in small bowl.
3 Spread half the mayonnaise mixture over each omelette; top with watercress, salmon, and cucumber. Roll omelette to enclose filling. Cut in half to serve, if you like.

Pack omelette wrap, wrapped in parchment, in lunchbox.

roast sweet potato and spinach frittata

This recipe is also nut-free.

2 medium sweet potatoes (28 oz)
1 tablespoon olive oil
2 teaspoons ground cumin
1¾ oz (about 1½ cups) baby spinach leaves,
    coarsely chopped
¼ cup (1 oz) finely grated parmesan cheese
6 eggs, beaten lightly
⅔ cup cream

1 Preheat oven to 350°F/325°F convection. Oil 6-hole (¾-cup) jumbo muffin pan; line bases with parchment.
2 Peel sweet potatoes; cut into ¼-inch slices. Combine potatoes, oil, and cumin in large, shallow baking dish; roast about 20 minutes or until tender. Cool 10 minutes.
3 Divide spinach, cheese, then potatoes among pan holes, finishing with potato.
4 Whisk egg and cream in medium bowl; pour into pan holes.
5 Bake about 25 minutes. Stand in pan 5 minutes; using small spatula, loosen frittatas from edge of pan before turning out, top-side up.

Pack frittata, lightly wrapped in parchment, in lunchbox.

omelette wrap

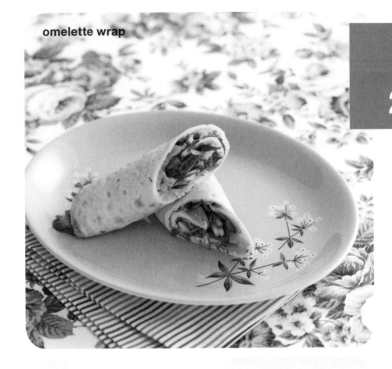

prep + cook time
15 minutes (+ cooling)
makes 2
nutritional count per
wrap 313 calories;
20.8 g total fat
(4.5 g saturated fat);
5.2 g carbohydrate;
1.4 g fiber;
25.9 g protein

prep + cook time
1 hour **makes 6**
nutritional count per
frittata 303 calories;
21 g total fat
(10.3 g saturated fat);
16.9 g carbohydrate;
2.3 g fiber;
10.8 g protein

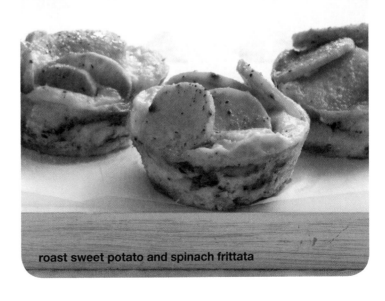

roast sweet potato and spinach frittata

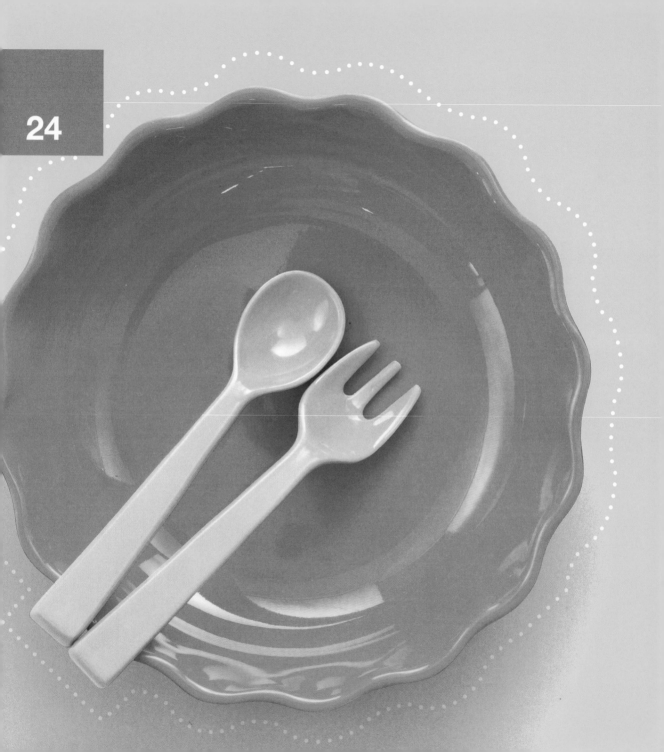

My favorite recipes

....

....

....

....

....

....

....

....

After-school snacks Refuel after a hard day with a muffin or brownie. Some of these recipes are also great lunchbox treats.

pancetta and cheese muffins

This recipe is also nut-free.

1 teaspoon olive oil
7 oz gluten-free pancetta,
finely chopped
4 scallions, thinly sliced
1¼ cups gluten-free
self-rising flour
⅓ cup polenta
¾ cup (3 oz) pizza cheese
⅔ cup milk
2 eggs
½ stick butter, melted

1 Preheat oven to 400°F/375°F convection. Line 12-hole (⅓-cup) muffin pan with paper liners.
2 Heat oil in medium frying pan over medium heat; cook pancetta, stirring, about 3 minutes, or until browned lightly. Add scallions; cook, stirring, until soft. Cool.
3 Combine flour, polenta, and ½ cup of the cheese in medium bowl; stir in combined milk and eggs, melted butter, and pancetta mixture.
4 Divide mixture among paper liners; sprinkle remaining cheese over. Bake about 20 minutes. Stand muffins in pan 5 minutes before turning, top-side up, onto wire rack to cool.

prep + cook time 35 minutes **makes** 12 **nutritional count per muffin** 143 calories; 9.7 g total fat (5.1 g saturated fat); 16.7 g carbohydrate; 0.4 g fiber; 7.2 g protein

My food notes

....

....

....

....

....

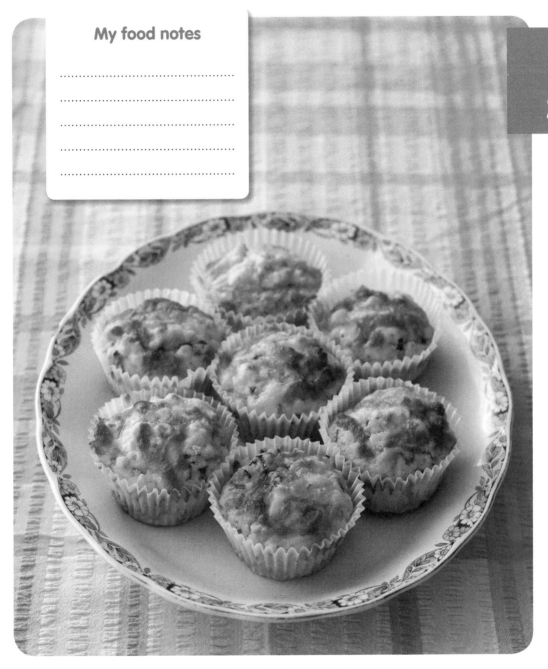

Did you know? Polenta is both ground corn and the name of a dish made with polenta. It comes in coarse and fine textures.

Allergy-free cooking for kids gluten-free After-school snacks

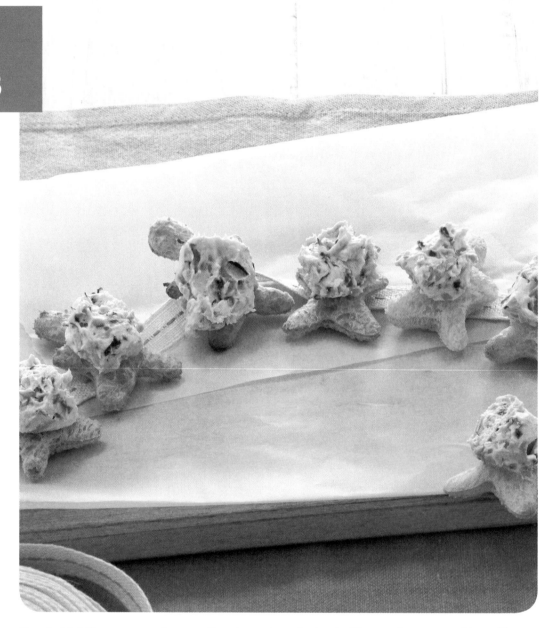

Handy hint You can use a larger cutter of any shape instead of the small cutter used here. The fillings will keep, covered, overnight in the fridge; use any leftover filling to make sandwiches for lunch the next day.

toastie men

This recipe is also egg-free and nut-free.

14 slices gluten-free white bread
14 slices gluten-free whole-wheat bread
9 oz spreadable cream cheese
2½ oz gluten-free thinly sliced ham, finely chopped
1 tablespoon finely chopped fresh chives
3 oz can tuna in springwater, drained
1 tablespoon finely chopped cornichons
1 tablespoon finely chopped fresh flat-leaf parsley

1 Preheat broiler.
2 Using gingerbread man cutter, cut three 2-inch men from each slice of bread; place on baking sheets. Toast bread, in batches, under broiler until browned both sides.
3 Divide cream cheese between two small bowls; stir ham and chives into one bowl, and stir tuna, cornichons, and parsley into remaining bowl.
4 Spread level teaspoons of ham mixture onto each white toast; spread level teaspoons of tuna mixture onto each whole-wheat toast.

Cornichon, French for gherkin, is a very small variety of pickled cucumber; they are available from delicatessens and most major supermarkets.

prep + cook time 45 minutes **makes** 42 of each **nutritional count per toastie man** 48 calories; 1.5 g total fat (0.7 g saturated fat); 6.3 g carbohydrate; 0.7 g fiber; 2.1 g protein

chocolate pecan cookies

1½ cups (6 oz) pecan pieces
1 stick butter, softened
½ cup superfine sugar
½ teaspoon vanilla extract
1 egg
⅔ cup brown rice flour
½ cup (100% corn) cornstarch
5 oz bittersweet chocolate, coarsely
   chopped
24 whole pecans
2 oz bittersweet chocolate, melted

1 Preheat oven to 350°F/325°F convection. Grease baking sheets; line with parchment.
2 Process pecan pieces until they are finely ground.
3 Beat butter, sugar, extract, and ground pecans in small bowl with electric mixer until light and fluffy. Add egg; beat until combined. Stir in sifted flours, then chopped chocolate.
4 Roll rounded tablespoons of mixture into balls; place 2½ inches apart on baking sheets, flatten slightly. Top with whole pecans.
5 Bake cookies about 20 minutes. Cool cookies on sheets, then drizzle melted chocolate over them.

prep + cook time 55 minutes (+ cooling) makes 24 nutritional count per cookie 186 calories; 12.8 g total fat (4.7 g saturated fat); 15.8 g carbohydrate; 0.8 g fiber; 1.8 g protein

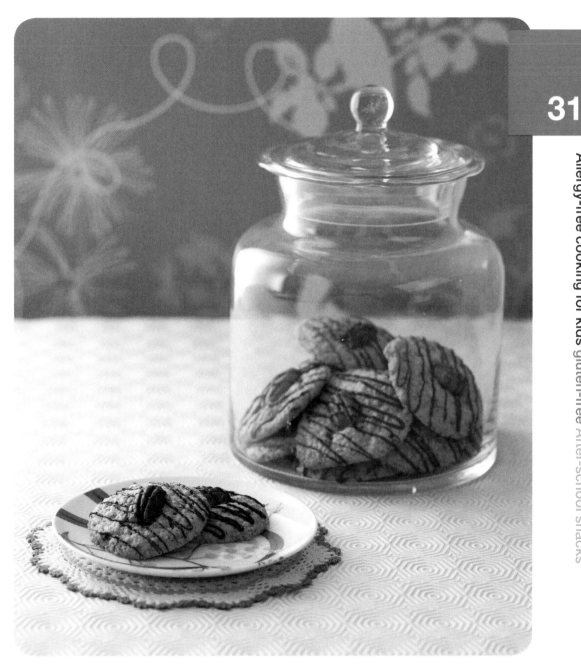

Healthy tip Brown rice flour retains the outer bran layer of the grain, which contains a valuable source of complex carbohydrates, vitamins, minerals, and fiber. It has a slightly chewy texture and nut-like flavor.

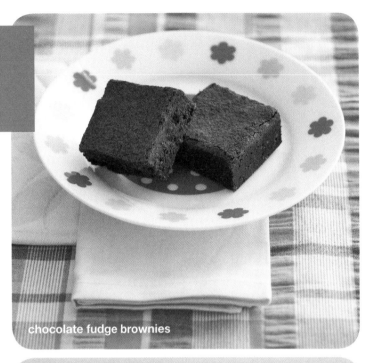

chocolate fudge brownies

prep + cook time
1 hour 10 minutes
(+ cooling) **makes** 18
**nutritional count per
brownie** 305 calories;
18 g total fat
(9.6 g saturated fat);
32 g carbohydrate;
0.8 g fiber;
3.6 g protein

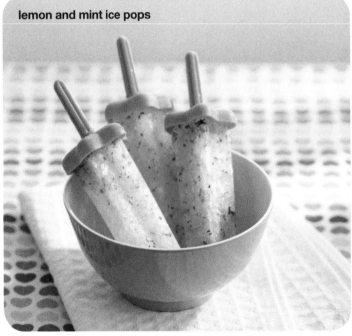

lemon and mint ice pops

prep + cook time
5 minutes (+ freezing)
**makes 4 nutritional
count per ice-pop**
42 calories;
0 g total fat
(0 g saturated fat);
10.3 g carbohydrate;
0 g fiber;
0.1 g protein

chocolate fudge brownies

1¼ sticks butter, coarsely chopped
10½ oz bittersweet chocolate,
   coarsely chopped
1½ cups firmly packed brown sugar
3 eggs
¾ cup (3 oz) ground hazelnuts
½ cup buckwheat flour
½ cup (4 oz) sour cream
¼ cup cocoa powder, sifted

1 Preheat oven to 350°F/325°F convection. Grease 7 x 11-inch baking pan; line base with parchment, extending paper 2 inches over long sides.
2 Melt butter and chocolate in medium saucepan over low heat. Add sugar; cook, stirring, 2 minutes. Cool mixture 10 minutes.
3 Stir in eggs, then ground nuts, flour, sour cream, and 2 tablespoons of the cocoa. Spread mixture into pan.
4 Bake brownies about 45 minutes. Cool in pan before cutting into squares. Dust with remaining sifted cocoa to serve.

lemon and mint ice pops

This recipe is also nut-free, dairy-free, and egg-free.

1½ cups lemonade
1 teaspoon finely grated lemon rind
1 tablespoon lemon juice
2 teaspoons finely chopped fresh mint

1 Combine lemonade, rind, juice, and mint in medium freezer-proof pitcher; freeze mixture about 1 hour or until partially frozen.
2 Stir mixture; pour into four ⅓ cup popsicle molds. Freeze overnight until firm.

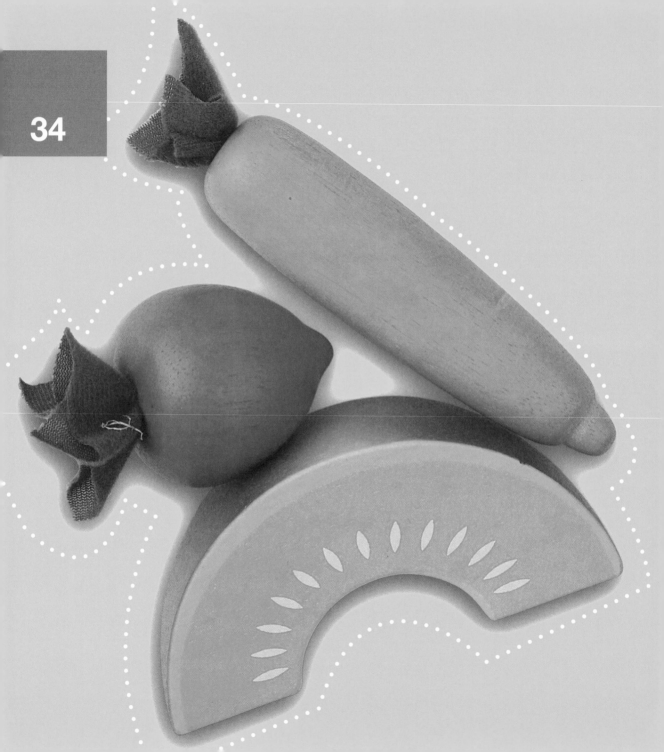

My favorite recipes

....
....
....
....
....
....
....
....

Dinner for everyone There's no need to cook separate meals for the family because everyone will enjoy these recipes.

egg, bacon, and parmesan pies

This recipe is also nut-free.

2 teaspoons vegetable oil
3 gluten-free bacon strips, finely chopped
1 small yellow onion (3 oz), finely chopped
1 clove garlic, crushed
4 eggs
¼ cup cream
¼ cup (1 oz) finely grated parmesan cheese
1 tablespoon finely chopped fresh chives
pastry
1 cup rice flour
¼ cup (100% corn) cornstarch
¼ cup soy flour
¼ cup finely grated parmesan cheese
1¼ sticks cold butter, chopped
2 tablespoons cold water, approximately

1 Make pastry.

2 Preheat oven to 425°F/400°F convection. Oil 6-hole (¾-cup) jumbo muffin pan.

3 Roll pastry between sheets of parchment until ¼-inch thick; cut six 4-inch rounds from pastry. Ease pastry rounds into pan holes, pressing into bases and sides; prick bases with fork.

4 Bake pastry shells about 10 minutes or until browned lightly. Cool shells in pan. Reduce oven temperature to 400°F/375°F convection.

5 Meanwhile, heat oil in small frying pan over medium heat; cook bacon, onion, and garlic, stirring, until bacon is soft. Divide bacon mixture among pastry shells.

6 Whisk eggs and cream in medium pitcher; stir in cheese and chives. Fill pastry shells with egg mixture. Bake about 25 minutes or until set.

pastry Process flours, cheese, and butter until fine. Add enough of the water to make ingredients come together. Cover; refrigerate 30 minutes.

prep + cook time 50 minutes (+ refrigeration and cooling) makes 6 nutritional count per pie
548 calories; 37.9 g total fat (20.8 g saturated fat); 54 g carbohydrate; 1.5 g fiber; 17.6 g protein

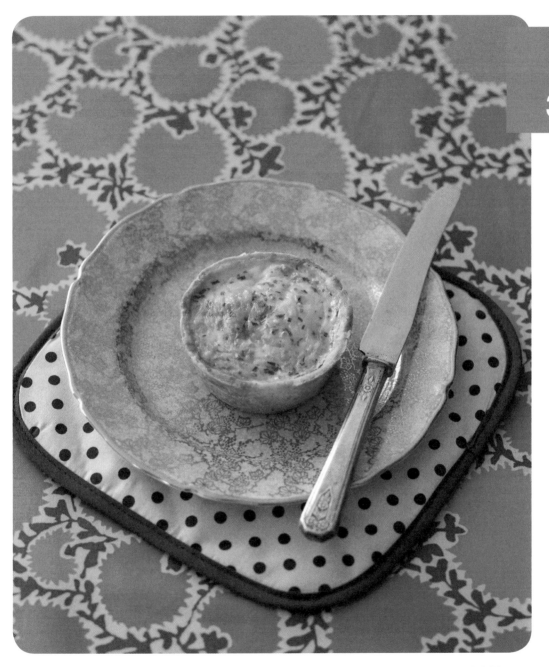

Handy hint You may have to make a double serving of this recipe, as hungry adults and children alike will be fighting for a taste. These would also make a great lunchbox or after-school treat.

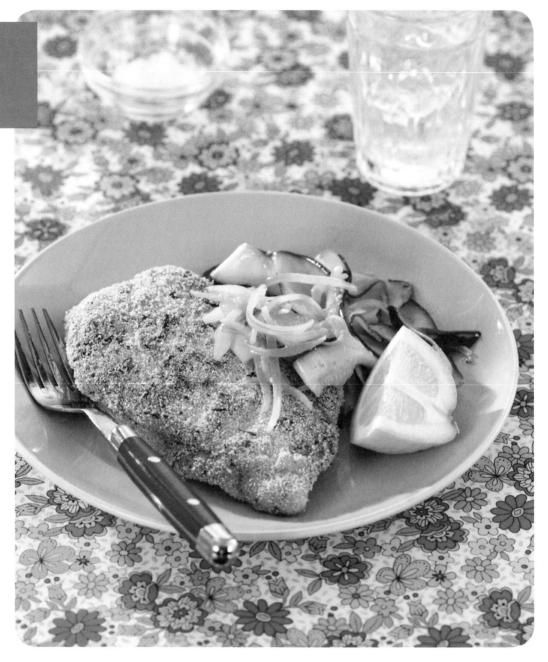

Did you know? Zucchini, sometimes called courgette, is a summer squash. Its color ranges from dark green to yellow. It's an excellent source of vitamin C, fiber, and folate.

polenta-coated chicken

This recipe is also nut-free.

4 chicken breast fillets (1¾ lbs)
¼ cup (100% corn) cornstarch
1 egg, beaten lightly
1 tablespoon gluten-free mayonnaise
1 tablespoon water
1¼ cups polenta
1 tablespoon finely chopped fresh oregano
    leaves
vegetable oil, for shallow-frying
lemon buttered zucchini
3 medium zucchini (13 oz)
½ stick butter
1 medium brown onion (5 oz), sliced
1 clove garlic, crushed
1½ tablespoons lemon juice

1 Place chicken between sheets of plastic wrap; gently pound until ⅓-inch thick. Toss chicken in cornstarch; shake off excess. Dip chicken into combined egg, mayonnaise, and water; then coat in combined polenta and oregano, pressing coating on firmly. Refrigerate chicken on baking sheet 10 minutes.

2 Make lemon buttered zucchini.

3 Heat vegetable oil in large frying pan over medium-high heat; shallow-fry chicken until browned lightly both sides and cooked through; drain on paper towels. Serve with lemon buttered zucchini.

lemon buttered zucchini Using vegetable peeler, cut zucchini into long strips. Melt butter in medium saucepan over medium heat; cook onion and garlic, stirring, until onion is soft. Add zucchini; cook, stirring, until zucchini is just soft, stir in juice. Cover to keep warm.

prep + cook time 30 minutes (+ refrigeration) serves 4 nutritional count per serving
1001 calories; 67.8 g total fat (18.3 g saturated fat); 48.5 g carbohydrate; 3.7 g fiber; 48.8 g protein

rice moussaka

This recipe is also nut-free.

1 large eggplant (18 oz)
2 tablespoons olive oil
1 clove garlic, crushed
3 scallions, finely chopped
3½ oz button mushrooms, thinly sliced
2 tablespoons water
14 oz can crushed tomatoes
2 teaspoons tomato paste
½ teaspoon ground cinnamon
1 teaspoon white sugar
2 tablespoons finely chopped fresh
   flat-leaf parsley
1½ cups cooked white short-grain rice
2 tablespoons finely grated parmesan
   cheese
½ teaspoon ground nutmeg
white sauce
½ stick butter
⅓ cup (100% corn) cornstarch
1⅓ cups milk
½ cup cream
2 tablespoons finely grated parmesan
   cheese
1 egg yolk

1 Cut eggplant into ¼-inch slices. Place eggplant in strainer, sprinkle salt over them; stand 30 minutes. Rinse eggplant under cold water; drain on paper towels.

2 Preheat broiler. Place eggplant slices on baking sheets; brush with half the oil. Broil both sides until browned lightly.

3 Preheat oven to 375°F/350°F convection. Grease 6-cup ovenproof baking dish.

4 Heat remaining oil in large saucepan over medium heat; cook garlic, onion, and mushrooms, stirring, until onion is soft. Add the water; cook, uncovered, until liquid has evaporated. Add undrained tomatoes, paste, cinnamon, sugar, and parsley; simmer, uncovered, until thickened slightly. Stir in rice and cheese.

5 Make white sauce.

6 Place one-third of the eggplant slices over base of prepared dish; top with half the rice mixture, then half the remaining eggplant, remaining rice mixture, and remaining eggplant. Spread white sauce over eggplant; sprinkle nutmeg over it. Bake moussaka about 30 minutes or until browned lightly.

white sauce Melt butter in medium saucepan over medium-low heat. Add cornstarch; cook, stirring, until mixture thickens and bubbles. Gradually stir in milk and cream; stir until sauce boils and thickens. Remove from heat; stir in cheese and egg yolk.

prep + cook time 1 hour (+ standing) serves 4 nutritional count per serving 733 calories; 42.8 g total fat (22.3 g saturated fat); 69.1 g carbohydrate; 5.6 g fiber; 14 g protein

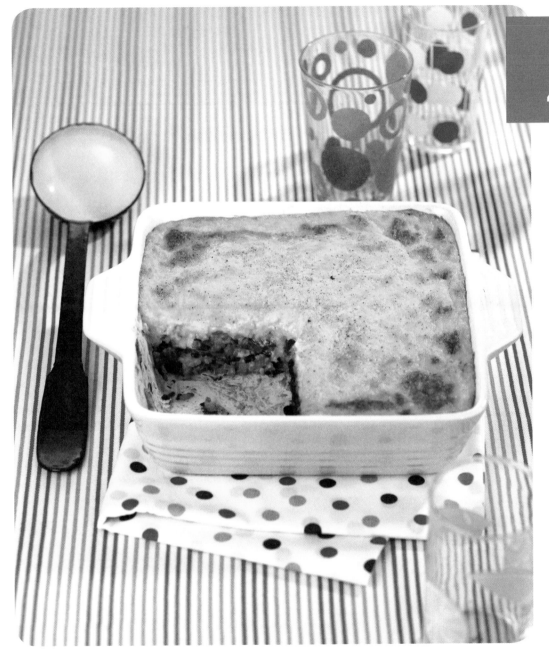

Handy hint You need to cook ½ cup white short-grain rice for this recipe. Short-grain rice is a fat, almost round grain with a high starch content, so the grains tend to clump together when cooked.

Allergy-free cooking for kids gluten-free Dinner for everyone

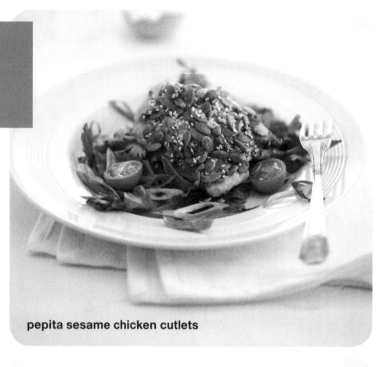

pepita sesame chicken cutlets

prep + cook time
1 hour 10 minutes
serves 4
nutritional count
per serving
369 calories;
21.9 g total fat
(4 g saturated fat);
2 g carbohydrate;
4.5 g fiber;
28.8 g protein

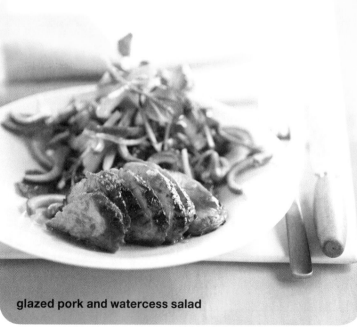

glazed pork and watercess salad

prep + cook time
30 minutes serves 4
nutritional count per
serving 451 calories;
14.1 g total fat
(3.2 g saturated fat);
29.9 g carbohydrate;
4.3 g fiber;
49.6 g protein

pepita sesame chicken cutlets

This recipe is also dairy-free.

1 tablespoon sesame seeds
⅓ cup pepitas (dried baby pumpkin seeds)
2 teaspoons finely grated lime rind
2 tablespoons lime juice
2 cloves garlic, crushed
4 chicken thigh cutlets (1¾ lbs)
1 egg white, beaten lightly
mint and parsley salad
1 tablespoon macadamia or vegetable oil
2 tablespoons lime juice
1 tablespoon non-alcoholic apple cider
   vinegar
1 cup firmly packed fresh flat-leaf parsley
   leaves
1 cup firmly packed fresh mint leaves
4 oz cherry tomatoes, halved
2 scallions, thinly sliced

1 Preheat oven to 400°F/375°F convection.
2 Combine seeds, pepitas, rind, juice, and garlic in small bowl.
3 Brush chicken all over with egg white; press seed mixture onto top side only. Place chicken on baking sheet, refrigerate, seeded-side up, 10 minutes. Cook, covered, 30 minutes. Uncover; cook 20 minutes, or until cooked through.
4 Make mint and parsley salad. Serve chicken with salad.
mint and parsley salad Whisk oil, juice, and vinegar in medium bowl. Add remaining ingredients; toss gently.

glazed pork and watercress salad

This recipe is also dairy-free and egg-free.

¼ cup honey
¼ cup tamarind concentrate
1¼ inch piece fresh ginger, grated
2 cloves garlic, crushed
1¾ lbs pork fillets
3½ oz watercress, trimmed
1 medium red onion (6 oz), thinly sliced
2 Lebanese cucumbers (9 oz), seeded,
   thinly sliced
1 medium yellow pepper (7 oz), thinly sliced
½ cup (3 oz) roasted unsalted cashews

1 Combine honey, tamarind, ginger, and garlic in small bowl. Combine pork with a third of the honey mixture in medium bowl.
2 Cook pork on heated oiled grill pan (or grill or barbecue) until browned all over and cooked as desired. Cover; stand 10 minutes, then thickly slice.
3 Meanwhile, combine remaining ingredients with half the remaining honey mixture in medium bowl.
4 Drizzle remaining honey mixture over pork; serve with salad.

beef lasagna

This recipe is also nut-free, dairy-free, and egg-free.

2 teaspoons olive oil
1 medium yellow onion (5 oz), finely chopped
1 stalk celery (5 oz), trimmed, finely chopped
1 small zucchini (3 oz), finely chopped
1 small carrot (2 oz), finely chopped
2 cloves garlic, crushed
1⅓ lbs ground beef
28 oz can crushed tomatoes
½ cup tomato paste
16 x 7 inch rice paper squares
1 tablespoon finely chopped fresh chives

white sauce
1½ cups water
1 cup gluten-free soy milk
2 cloves
1 dried bay leaf
2 tablespoons dairy-free spread
2 tablespoons (100% corn) cornstarch
3½ oz chive-flavored soy cheese, coarsely chopped

1 Heat oil in large frying pan over medium heat; cook onion, celery, zucchini, carrot, and garlic, stirring, until onion is soft. Add beef; cook, stirring, until browned. Add undrained tomatoes and paste; cook, stirring, about 10 minutes, or until sauce thickens slightly.

2 Meanwhile, make white sauce.

3 Preheat oven to 375°F/350°F convection. Oil deep 2½-quart rectangular ovenproof dish.

4 Dip eight rice paper squares, one at a time, into bowl of warm water until soft; place on board covered with a towel. Spread 1½ cups beef mixture over base of dish; top with softened rice paper sheets. Top with half of the remaining beef mixture and half of the white sauce.

5 Soften remaining rice paper, place on top of beef mixture; top with remaining beef mixture and white sauce.

6 Bake lasagna, uncovered, about 50 minutes, or until lightly browned. Stand 10 minutes; garnish with chives before serving.

white sauce Combine the water, milk, cloves, and bay leaf in medium saucepan; bring to the boil. Strain milk mixture into large heatproof pitcher; discard solids. Melt spread in same saucepan; add cornstarch, cook, stirring 1 minute. Gradually add hot milk mixture, stirring, constantly, until mixture boils and thickens. Stir in cheese.

prep + cook time 1 hour 30 minutes serves 6 nutritional count per serving 355 calories; 15.2 g total fat (4.2 g saturated fat); 26.9 g carbohydrate; 4.5 g fiber; 25.3 g protein

My food notes

....

....

....

....

....

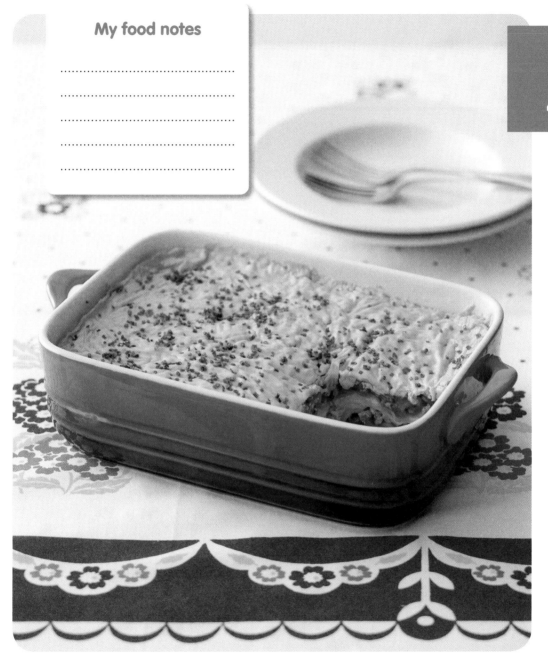

Handy hint If you don't have an intolerance to milk products you can substitute 2½ cups cow's milk for the soy milk and water in the white sauce recipe, and butter for the dairy-free spread.

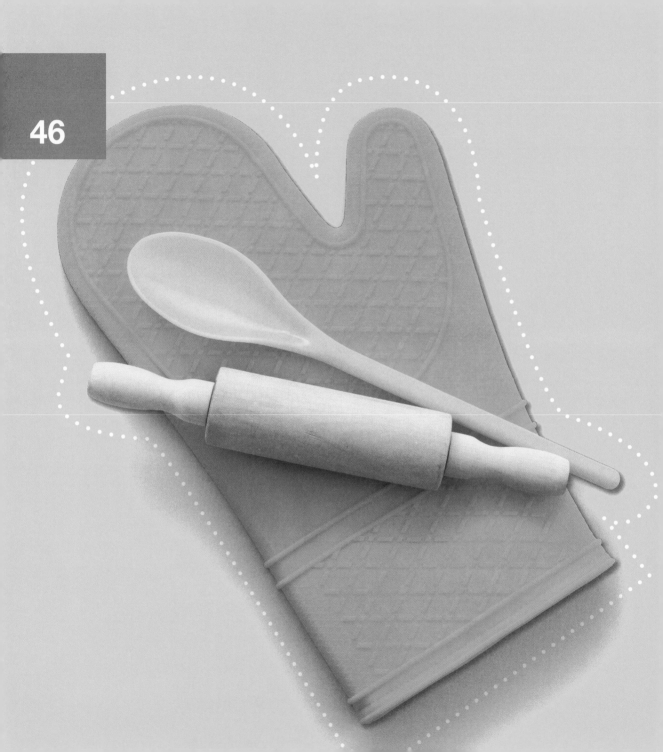

My favorite recipes

....

....

....

....

....

....

....

....

Seriously sweet Chocolate nut cake, custard tarts, cheesecake, and berry crumbles—who said sweets were off the menu?

chocolate strawberry tart

⅓ cup strawberry jam
⅔ cup cream
2 tablespoons unsalted butter
7 oz bittersweet chocolate, finely chopped
6 strawberries, halved
hazelnut crust
1½ cups (5 oz) ground hazelnuts
⅓ cup superfine sugar
¼ cup (100% corn) cornstarch
1 stick cold unsalted butter, chopped
1 egg yolk

1 Make hazelnut crust.
2 Grease 9-inch removable bottom tart pan. Roll hazelnut dough between sheets of parchment until large enough to line pan. Ease dough into pan, press into base and side; trim edge. Cover; refrigerate 30 minutes.
3 Preheat oven to 400°F/375°F convection.
4 Place tart pan on baking sheet. Bake hazelnut crust about 25 minutes. Spread jam over crust; return to oven 2 minutes. Remove from oven; cool.
5 Heat cream in medium saucepan; remove from heat, stir in butter and chocolate, then whisk until smooth. Pour chocolate mixture into crust; refrigerate 2 hours. Top tart with strawberries to serve.
hazelnut crust Process ground nuts, sugar, cornstarch, and butter until crumbly; add egg yolk, pulse until mixture comes together. Knead dough gently on floured surface until smooth. Wrap in plastic; refrigerate 1 hour.

prep + cook time 50 minutes (+ refrigeration) **serves** 12 **nutritional count per serving** 382 calories; 29.1 g total fat (14 g saturated fat); 26.6 g carbohydrate; 1.8 g fiber; 3.4 g protein

My food notes

....
....
....
....
....

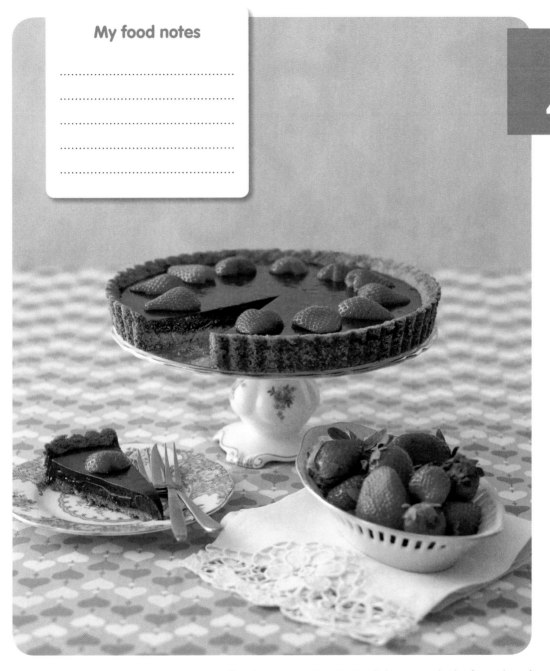

Heathy tip Hazelnuts are rich in vitamin E, a fat-soluble vitamin that is important in the formation of healthy red blood cells. It's also an antioxidant, which protects the body from tissue and cellular damage.

My food notes

....

....

....

....

....

....

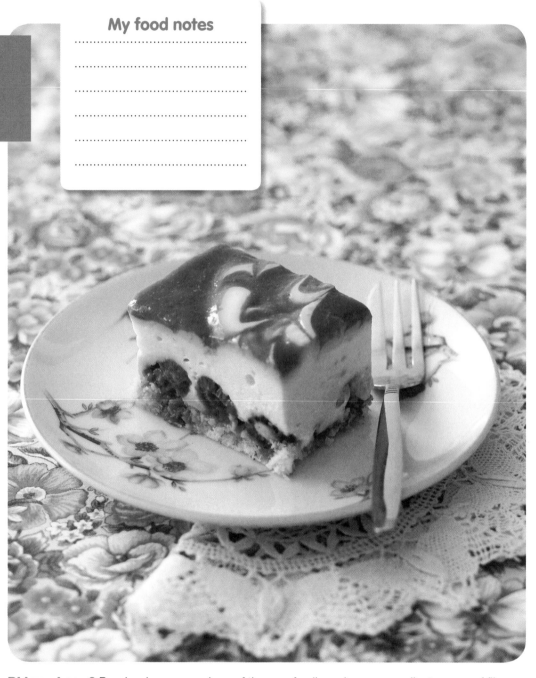

Did you know? Raspberries are members of the rose family and are an excellent source of fiber and vitamin C; they also contain iron and folate. Other berries can be used instead.

raspberry cheesecake

2 egg whites
¾ cup desiccated (dried) coconut
¾ cup shredded coconut
⅓ cup superfine sugar
3 teaspoons powdered gelatin
¼ cup water
18 oz cream cheese, softened
½ cup superfine sugar, extra
1¼ cups cream
1 teaspoon vanilla extract
10½ oz raspberries

1 Preheat oven to 350°F/325°F convection. Grease deep 7-inch-square cake pan; line base and sides with parchment, extending paper 2 inches over sides.
2 Beat egg whites lightly in medium bowl, stir in coconut and sugar; press mixture firmly over base of pan. Bake base 15 minutes or until browned lightly. Cool.
3 Meanwhile, sprinkle gelatin over the water in small heatproof bowl; stand bowl in small saucepan of simmering water. Stir until gelatin dissolves. Cool 5 minutes.
4 Beat cream cheese and extra sugar in medium bowl with electric mixer until smooth; beat in cream and extract. Stir in gelatin mixture.
5 Sprinkle half the raspberries over coconut base; pour in filling. Blend or process remaining raspberries; strain. Drizzle raspberry puree over filling; pull skewer backward and forward several times for marbled effect. Refrigerate 3 hours or overnight.

Allergy-free cooking for kids gluten-free Seriously sweet

prep + cook time 35 minutes (+ refrigeration) serves 12 nutritional count per serving
384 calories; 31.2 g total fat (21.7 g saturated fat); 19.4 g carbohydrate; 2.8 g fiber; 6 g protein

coconut custard tarts

1½ cups desiccated (dried) coconut
1½ cups shredded coconut
⅔ cup superfine sugar
4 egg whites, beaten lightly
3 egg yolks
½ cup superfine sugar, extra
1 tablespoon arrowroot
¾ cup milk
½ cup cream
1 vanilla bean
2-inch strip lemon rind
1 tablespoon confectioners' sugar

1 Preheat oven to 350°F/325°F convection. Grease 12-hole (⅓-cup) muffin pan.

2 Combine coconut and sugar in large bowl; stir in egg whites. Press mixture over base and side of pan holes to make tart shells.

3 Whisk egg yolks, extra sugar, and arrowroot together in medium saucepan; gradually whisk in milk and cream to make custard.

4 Split vanilla bean in half lengthwise; scrape seeds into custard, discard pod. Add lemon rind to custard; stir over medium heat until mixture boils and thickens slightly. Remove from heat immediately; discard rind.

5 Spoon warm custard into pastry shells; bake about 15 minutes or until set and browned lightly. Stand tarts in pan 10 minutes. Transfer to wire rack to cool. Dust tarts with sifted confectioners' sugar to serve.

prep + cook time 45 minutes **makes** 12 **nutritional count per tart** 295 calories; 19.3 g total fat (15.1 g saturated fat); 25.4 g carbohydrate; 2.9 g fiber; 3.9 g protein

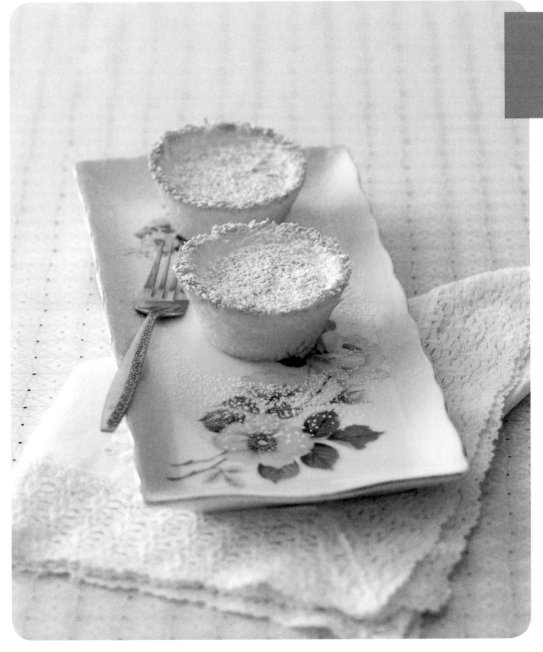

Did you know? Arrowroot is an easily digestible almost pure-starch substance from the fleshy root of a West Indian plant. It is used to produce clear thickened sauces when added to hot liquids.

Allergy-free cooking for kids gluten-free Seriously sweet

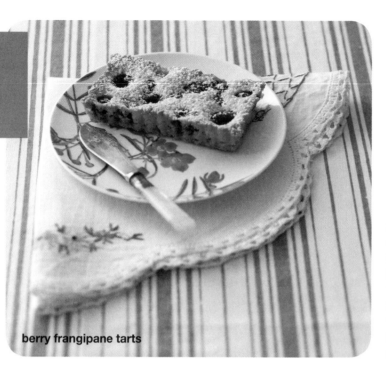

berry frangipane tarts

prep + cook time
45 minutes makes 6
nutritional count per
tart 271 calories;
19.5 g total fat
(7.6 g saturated fat);
18.8 g carbohydrate;
2.2 g fiber;
4.4 g protein

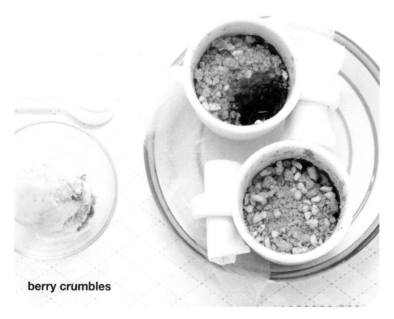

berry crumbles

prep + cook time
50 minutes makes 4
nutritional count per
crumble 218 calories;
8.2 g total fat
(5.2 g saturated fat);
31.2 g carbohydrate;
2.2 g fiber;
3.5 g protein

berry frangipane tarts

5 tablespoons butter, softened
½ teaspoon vanilla extract
⅓ cup superfine sugar
1 egg
¾ cup (3 oz) ground almonds
1 tablespoon (100% corn) cornstarch
5 oz (about 1 cup) fresh blueberries and raspberries
1 tablespoon confectioners' sugar

1 Preheat oven to 350°F/325°F convection. Grease six 2 x 4-inch removable bottom tart pans; place on baking sheet.
2 Beat butter, extract, and superfine sugar in small bowl with electric mixer until light and fluffy. Add egg; beat until combined. Stir in nuts and cornstarch. Spoon mixture into pans; smooth surface, sprinkle berries over.
3 Bake tarts about 30 minutes. Stand in pans 10 minutes before carefully turning, top-side up, onto parchment-covered wire rack.
4 Serve tarts warm or cold, dusted with sifted confectioners' sugar.

berry crumbles

This recipe is also nut-free and egg-free.

2 cups (10½ oz) fresh or frozen mixed berries
4 tablespoons strawberry-flavored frozen yogurt
crumble topping
4 tablespoons puffed rice
2 tablespoons gluten-free all-purpose flour
2 tablespoons brown rice flour
2 tablespoons brown sugar
2 tablespoons butter

1 Preheat oven to 400°F/375°F convection. Grease four ¾-cup ovenproof dishes.
2 Make crumble topping.
3 Divide berries into dishes; sprinkle crumble topping over each. Bake about 30 minutes or until browned lightly.
4 Serve crumbles warm with the frozen yogurt.
crumble topping Blend or process puffed rice until fine. Add flours, sugar, and butter; process until crumbly.

carrot cupcakes

This recipe is also nut-free.

⅔ cup firmly packed brown sugar

½ cup vegetable oil

2 eggs

1½ cups (8 oz) firmly packed coarsely grated
carrot (see handy hint, page 57)

½ cup potato flour

¼ cup (100% corn) cornstarch

¼ cup rice flour

1 teaspoon gluten-free baking powder

¼ teaspoon baking soda

1 teaspoon pie spice

½ cup confectioners' sugar

9 oz gluten-free white fondant

yellow, green, and pink food coloring

gluten-free sprinkles

butter cream

7 tablespoons butter, softened

1 cup confectioners' sugar

1½ tablespoons milk

1 Preheat oven to 350°F/325°F convection.
Line 12-hole (⅓-cup) muffin pan with liners.
2 Beat sugar, oil, and eggs in bowl with
mixer until thick and creamy. Transfer
mixture to large bowl; stir in carrot, then
sifted dry ingredients. Divide mixture among
liners.
3 Bake cupcakes about 20 minutes. Stand
cupcakes in pan 5 minutes; turn, top-side
up, onto wire rack to cool.
4 Make butter cream.
5 Divide butter cream equally into three
small bowls; tint each bowl with one of the
colors: green, pink, and yellow. Spread each
color butter cream over four cakes.
6 On a surface dusted with sifted
confectioners' sugar, knead the fondant until
smooth. Divide icing into three equal
portions; tint each portion with one of the
colors: yellow, green, and pink. Roll each
portion until ⅛ inch thick.
7 Cut four 1¾-inch rounds from each icing
portion. Cut each round in half for the
cupcake "tops." Using picture as a guide,
position "tops" on cakes.
8 Working with one icing portion at a time,
use a fluted pastry wheel to cut a 1 x 7-inch
strip from yellow, green, and pink icings. Cut
four cupcake cup "bases" from each strip of
icing. Mark vertical lines on each of the
"bases." Position "bases" on cakes.
9 Brush a tiny amount of water onto tops of
the cupcake "tops"; decorate with sprinkles.
butter cream Beat butter in small bowl with
electric mixer until fluffy; gradually beat in
sifted confectioners' sugar, then the milk.

prep + cook time 1 hour 15 minutes (+ cooling) makes 12 nutritional count per cupcake
480 calories; 21 g total fat (8.3 g saturated fat); 70.1 g carbohydrate; 0.8 g fiber; 2 g protein

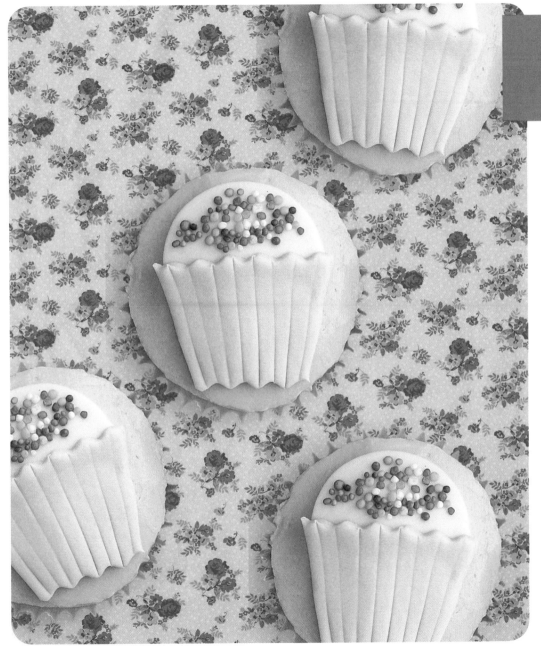

Handy hints You will need about 3 medium carrots (12 oz) for this recipe. Gluten-free sprinkles are available in the specialty baking stores and online.

Allergy-free cooking for kids gluten-free Seriously sweet

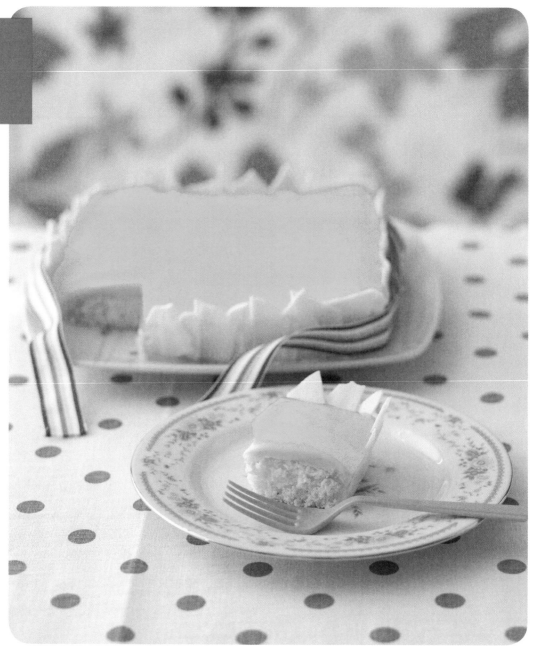

Did you know? White chocolate is not considered real chocolate because it does not have chocolate liquor, which comes from the finely ground nib (center) of the cocoa bean.

pineapple and white chocolate jelly cake

This recipe is also nut-free.

1 teaspoon vegetable oil
3 oz packet pineapple gelatin
3 eggs
½ cup superfine sugar
¾ cup (100% corn) cornstarch
5 oz white chocolate, melted
3 ft ribbon
white chocolate ganache
1¼ cups cream
13 oz white chocolate, coarsely chopped

1 Oil deep 7-inch square cake pan. Make gelatin according to packet directions; pour into pan. Refrigerate 3 hours or until set.

2 Make white chocolate ganache; cool.

3 Pour three-quarters of ganache over the gelatin; refrigerate 1 hour.

4 Meanwhile, preheat oven to 350°F/325°F convection. Grease 9-inch-square cake pan; line base with parchment.

5 Beat eggs in small bowl with electric mixer until thick and creamy. Gradually beat in sugar until dissolved. Fold in triple-sifted cornstarch. Spread mixture into pan.

6 Bake cake about 20 minutes. Turn cake onto parchment-covered wire rack to cool.

7 Trim cake to 7-inch square; place in pan on top of ganache and jelly. Refrigerate 30 minutes.

8 Meanwhile, spread chocolate onto parchment-lined tray until ⅛-inch thick; refrigerate about 10 minutes or until set. Break into small pieces.

9 Place base of pan in sink of hot water for a few seconds to loosen gelatin; quickly invert cake onto serving plate. Secure chocolate pieces around edges of cake with remaining ganache; secure ribbon.

white chocolate ganache Stir cream and chocolate in medium heatproof bowl over medium saucepan of simmering water until smooth (do not let water touch base of bowl). Cool.

prep + cook time 40 minutes (+ refrigeration) serves 16 nutritional count per serving
338 calories; 20 g total fat (12.4 g saturated fat); 35.4 g carbohydrate; 0 g fiber; 4.3 g protein

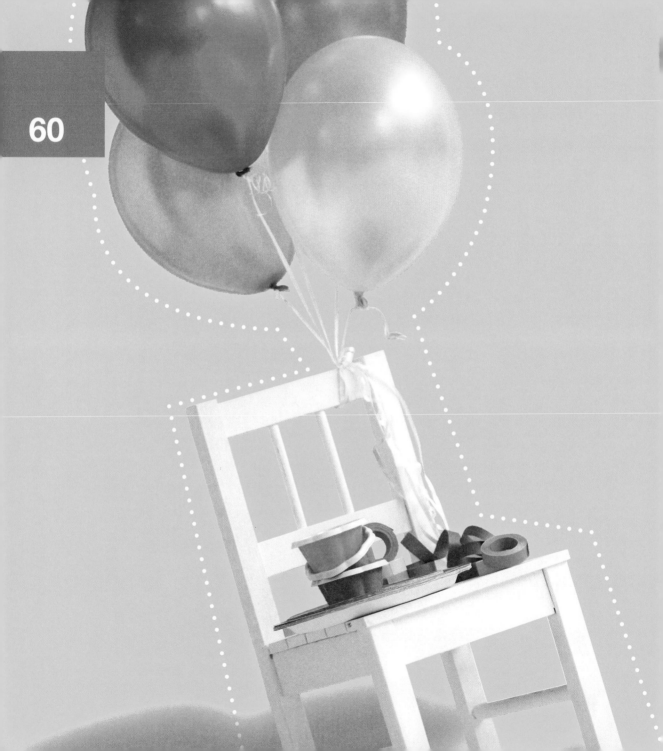

My favorite recipes

....
....
....
....
....
....
....
....
....

Party time Just like "real" party food, these gluten-free treats are just as delicious and just as much fun to eat.

mini meat pies

This recipe is also nut-free.

2 teaspoons vegetable oil
1 medium yellow onion (5 oz), finely
    chopped
2 gluten-free bacon strips, finely
    chopped
12 oz ground beef
2 tablespoons tomato paste
¼ cup arrowroot
2 cups gluten-free beef stock
1 egg, beaten lightly
pastry
1¾ cups rice flour
⅓ cup (100% corn) cornstarch
⅓ cup soy flour
1¾ sticks cold butter, chopped
¼ cup cold water, approximately

1 Heat oil in medium saucepan over medium heat; cook onion and bacon, stirring, until onion softens and bacon is browned. Add beef; cook, stirring, until browned.

2 Add paste and blended arrowroot and stock to pan; bring to the boil, stirring. Reduce heat; simmer, uncovered, until thickened. Cool.
3 Meanwhile, make pastry.
4 Preheat oven to 425°F/400°F convection. Oil twelve ¼-cup foil pie tins (2¾-inch top, 2-inch base); place on baking sheet.
5 Roll pastry between sheets of parchment until ¼ inch thick; cut twelve 3½-inch rounds from pastry. Ease pastry rounds into pie tins; press into base and sides. Spoon beef mixture into pastry shells; brush edges with egg. Cut twelve 2¾-inch rounds from remaining pastry; place rounds on pies, press to seal edges. Brush pies with egg; cut two small slits into top of each pie.
6 Bake pies about 25 minutes. Serve with gluten-free tomato sauce.
pastry Process flours and butter until mixture is fine. Add enough of the water to make ingredients come together. Cover; refrigerate 30 minutes.

prep + cook time 1 hour (+ refrigeration) makes 12 nutritional count per pie 247 calories;
19.3 g total fat (11 g saturated fat); 7.8 g carbohydrate; 0.7 g fiber; 10.7 g protein

My food notes

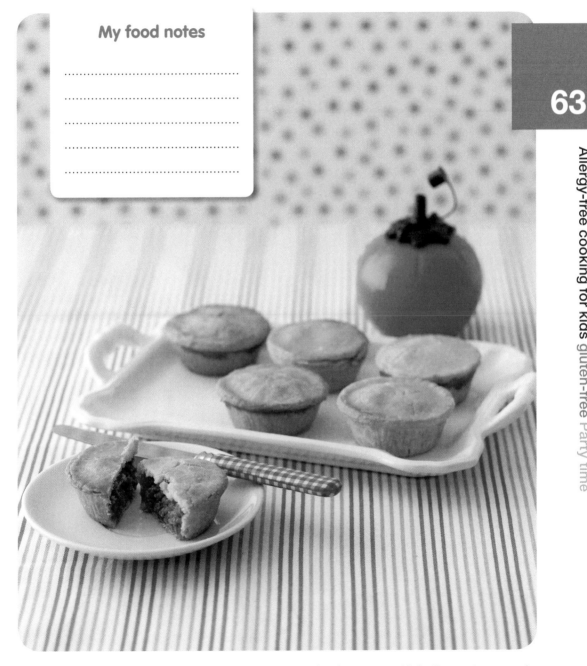

Handy hint These pies are good for lunchbox or after-school treats, too. Make them using ground pork and veal, ground chicken, or ground turkey and use a gluten-free chicken stock.

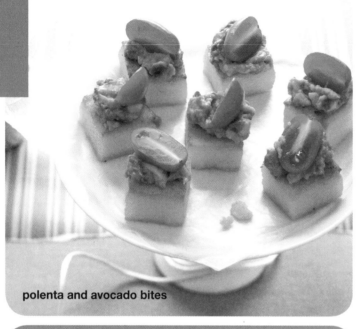

polenta and avocado bites

prep + cook time
35 minutes
(+ refrigeration)
makes 36
nutritional count per
piece 33 calories;
2.2 g total fat
(0.7 g saturated fat);
2.4 g carbohydrate;
0.2 g fiber;
0.8 g protein

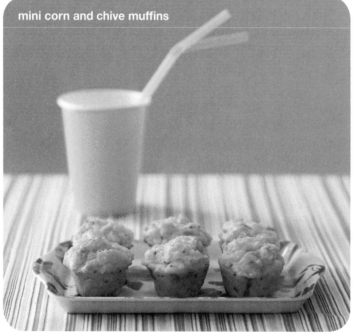

mini corn and chive muffins

prep + cook time
30 minutes
makes 24
nutritional count per
muffin 56 calories;
4.1 g total fat
(2.5 g saturated fat);
8.1 g carbohydrate;
0.5 g fiber;
1.5 g protein

polenta and avocado bites

This recipe is also nut-free and egg-free.

3 cups water
¾ cup polenta
½ cup (2 oz) coarsely grated
  cheddar cheese
1 medium avocado
2 teaspoons lemon juice
1 tablespoon olive oil
18 grape tomatoes, halved

1 Oil deep 8-inch-square cake pan.
2 Place the water in medium saucepan; bring to the boil. Gradually stir polenta into the water. Simmer, stirring, about 10 minutes, or until polenta thickens. Stir in cheese; spread polenta into pan, cool polenta 10 minutes. Cover polenta; refrigerate 1 hour, or until firm.
3 Mash avocado and juice in small bowl until mixture is almost smooth.
4 Invert polenta onto board; cut polenta into 36 squares. Heat oil in large frying pan over medium heat; cook polenta, turning, until browned all over.
5 Top polenta squares with avocado mixture, then tomatoes.

mini corn and chive muffins

This recipe is also nut-free.

1¼ cups gluten-free self-rising flour
6 tablespoons butter, melted
2 eggs, beaten lightly
2 4 oz cans gluten-free creamed corn
½ cup (2 oz) pizza cheese
2 tablespoons finely chopped fresh chives

1 Preheat oven to 400°F/375°F convection. Oil two 12-hole (1 tablespoon) mini muffin pans.
2 Sift flour into medium bowl; stir in butter, eggs, corn, cheese, and chives. Divide mixture among pan holes.
3 Bake muffins about 15 minutes. Stand muffins in pan 5 minutes before turning, top-side up, onto wire rack to cool.

mini pizza squares

This recipe is also nut-free.

13 oz packet gluten-free bread mix
⅓ cup tomato paste
2 medium tomatoes (2 lbs), thinly sliced
9 oz jar roasted peppers in oil, drained, coarsely chopped
½ small red onion (2 oz), sliced thinly
5 oz soft feta cheese, crumbled
15 oz can pineapple pieces, drained
3½ oz thinly sliced gluten-free ham, coarsely chopped
1 cup (3½ oz) pizza cheese
½ cup (2 oz) pitted green olives, halved
20 small fresh basil leaves
5 cherry tomatoes, quartered
20 fresh oregano leaves

1 Preheat oven to 425°F/400°F convection. Oil two 9 x 13-inch jelly roll pans; line bases with parchment, extending paper 2 inches over long sides.
2 Make bread mix according to packet directions; spread mixture into pans. Bake about 12 minutes or until browned lightly. Remove from oven.
3 Spread paste over crusts. Sprinkle sliced tomato, peppers, onion, and feta over one pizza crust. Sprinkle pineapple, ham, and pizza cheese over remaining pizza crust.
4 Bake pizzas about 15 minutes or until cheese melts and crusts are crisp. Cut each pizza into 20 squares. Top each peppers and feta pizza square with olives and basil leaves. Top each ham and pineapple pizza square with a tomato quarter and an oregano leaf.

prep + cook time 50 minutes makes 40 squares (20 of each pizza) nutritional count per pepper and feta pizza square 68 calories; 2.5 g total fat (1.2 g saturated fat); 8.3 g carbohydrate; 0.7 g fiber; 2.8 g protein nutritional count per ham and pineapple pizza square 65 calories; 1.4 g total fat (0.8 g saturated fat); 9.1 g carbohydrate; 0.8 g fiber; 3.6 g protein

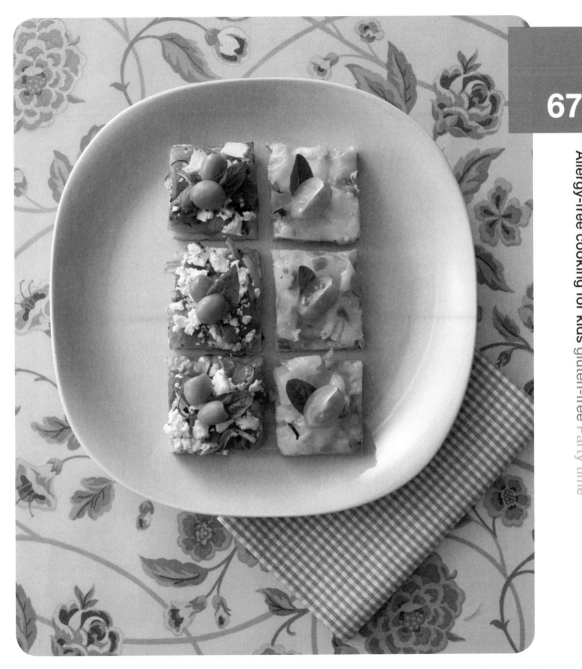

Handy hint These days gluten-free bread mixes are readily available from most supermarkets as well as health-food stores. The mixes are available in plain and whole-wheat; we used plain in this recipe.

toffee-on-a-stick

This recipe is also nut-free, dairy-free, and egg-free.

6 wooden popsicle sticks
1½ cups superfine sugar
½ cup water
1 tablespoon white vinegar
gluten-free sprinkles

1 Grease 12-hole (1 tablespoon) mini muffin pan. Cut popsicle sticks in half crosswise.

2 Combine sugar, water, and vinegar in medium heavy-based saucepan. Stir over heat, without boiling, until sugar is dissolved.

3 Bring mixture to the boil; boil, uncovered, without stirring, about 15 minutes, or until a small amount of sugar syrup "cracks" when dropped into a cup of cold water and sugar has turned light golden brown.

4 Remove from heat; allow bubbles to subside. Pour toffee mixture into prepared pan holes; scatter sprinkles over the top.

5 Stand toffees about 10 minutes; place sticks, cut-side down, into center of toffees. Stand toffees at room temperature until set.

prep + cook time 30 minutes (+ standing) makes 12 nutritional count per toffee 127 calories; 0 g total fat (0 g saturated fat); 31.2 g carbohydrate; 0 g fiber, 0 g protein

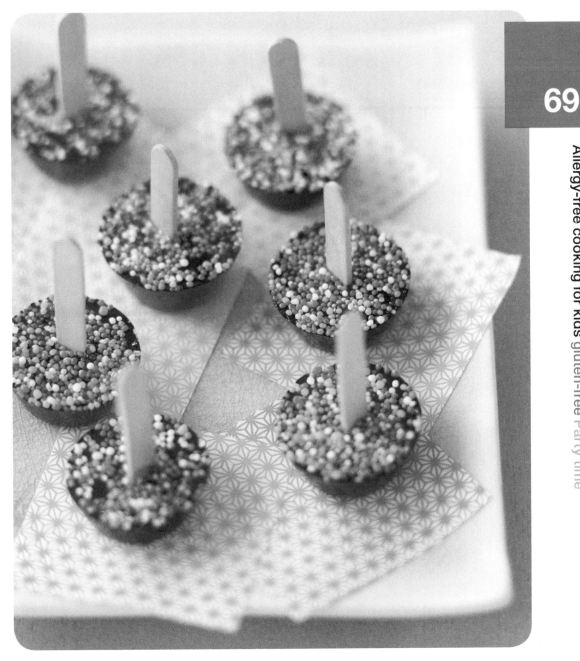

Handy hints Popsicle sticks are available from craft and hobby shops. For easy pouring, use a saucepan with a pouring lip, or carefully transfer the hot toffee to a heatproof pitcher.

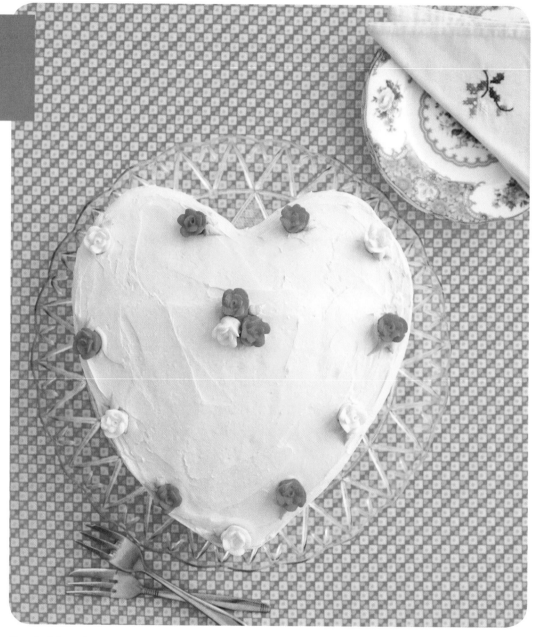

Handy hints For a dairy-free version of this cake, substitute dairy-free spread for the butter and soy milk for the milk. If you can't find gluten-free edible roses, use a rose piping tip to pipe on some of the frosting.

buttercake

This recipe is also nut-free.

1¾ sticks butter, softened
2¼ cups gluten-free self-rising flour
1 cup superfine sugar
½ cup milk
2 eggs
2 egg whites
about 1 dozen small gluten-free edible
    sugar roses
fluffy frosting
1 cup superfine sugar
½ cup water
2 egg whites
green and pink food coloring

1 Preheat oven to 350°F/325°F convection. Grease and line deep 10-inch heart-shaped cake pan.
2 Beat butter in medium bowl with electric mixer until lightened in color. Sift flour and ¼ cup of the sugar together. Beat flour mixture and milk into the butter, in two batches, only until combined.
3 Beat eggs and egg whites in small bowl with electric mixer until thick and creamy. Gradually add remaining sugar, one tablespoon at a time, beating until sugar dissolves between additions. With motor operating on low speed, gradually pour egg mixture into flour mixture; beat only until combined.
4 Spread mixture into pan; bake about 50 minutes. Stand cake 10 minutes; invert onto wire rack to cool.
5 Make fluffy frosting. Cover top and sides of cake with pink fluffy frosting; decorate cake with roses. Spoon green fluffy frosting into small piping bag with small plain tip; pipe leaves onto cake.

fluffy frosting Stir sugar and the water in small saucepan over heat, without boiling, until sugar is dissolved. Boil, uncovered, without stirring, about 5 minutes or until syrup reaches 240°F on a candy thermometer (syrup should be thick but not colored). Remove from heat; allow bubbles to subside. Beat egg whites in small bowl with electric mixer until soft peaks form. While mixer is operating, add hot syrup in a thin stream; beat on high speed about 10 minutes or until mixture is thick and cool. Transfer 2 tablespoons of the frosting to small bowl; tint green. Tint remaining frosting pink.

prep + cook time 1 hour 15 minutes serves 12 nutritional count per serving 325 calories; 15.1 g total fat (9.5 g saturated fat); 61.4 g carbohydrate; 0.4 g fiber; 3.1 g protein

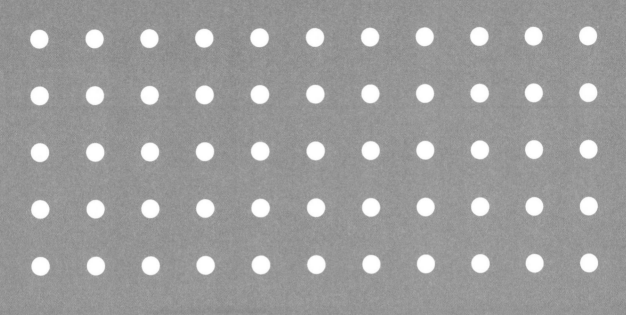

Dairy-free

There are many dairy substitutes available these days, including ice cream, popsicles, and sorbets.

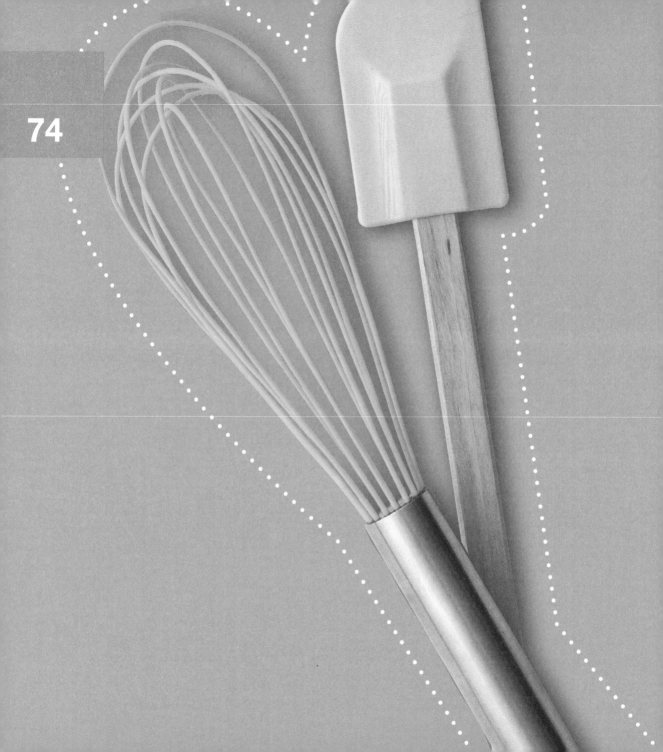

My favorite recipes

....

....

....

....

....

....

....

....

....

Breakfast The most important meal of the day—after all, it's been at least 8 hours since you last ate, so it's time to refuel.

mushroom and parsley omelette

This recipe is also nut-free and gluten-free.

4 eggs, beaten lightly
6 egg whites
17 oz cremini mushrooms, thinly sliced
⅓ cup loosely packed, coarsely chopped
   fresh flat-leaf parsley

1 Whisk beaten eggs with egg whites in medium bowl.
2 Spray an 8-inch frying pan with cooking spray; heat over medium. Cook the mushrooms, stirring, until tender. Combine mushrooms and parsley in small bowl.
3 Return pan to heat, add a quarter of the egg mixture; cook over medium heat, tilting pan, until almost set. Place a quarter of the mushroom mixture evenly over half of the omelette; fold omelette over to enclose filling, slide onto serving plate. Repeat with remaining egg and mushroom mixture to make a total of four omelettes.
4 Serve omelettes with thick slices of toasted sourdough, if you'd like.

oatmeal with poached pears and blueberries

This recipe is also nut-free and egg-free.

¾ cup hot water
⅓ cup rolled oats
1 small pear (6 oz), cored, coarsely chopped
½ cup cold water
2 tablespoons blueberries

1 Combine the hot water and oats in small saucepan over medium heat; cook, stirring, about 5 minutes, or until oatmeal is thick and creamy.
2 Place pear and the cold water in small saucepan; bring to the boil. Reduce heat, simmer, uncovered, about 5 minutes, or until pear softens.
3 Serve oatmeal topped with pears and 1 tablespoon of the poaching liquid; garnish with berries.

mushroom and parsley omelette

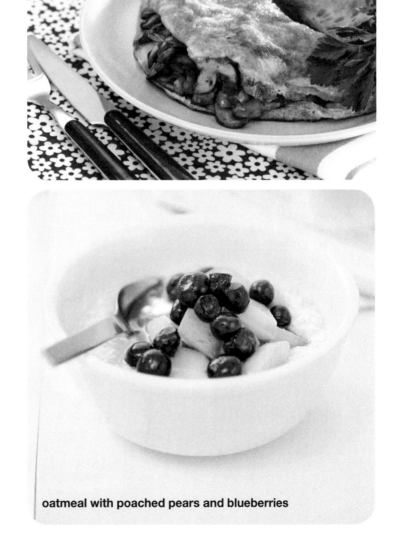

prep + cook time
20 minutes
serves 4
nutritional count
per serving
127 calories;
5.6 g total fat
(1.6 g saturated fat);
0.7 g carbohydrate;
3.4 g fiber;
16.6 g protein

prep + cook time
20 minutes
serves 1
nutritional count per
serving 211 calories;
2.7 g total fat
(0.5 g saturated fat);
43.4 g carbohydrate;
6.6 g fiber;
3.9 g protein

oatmeal with poached pears and blueberries

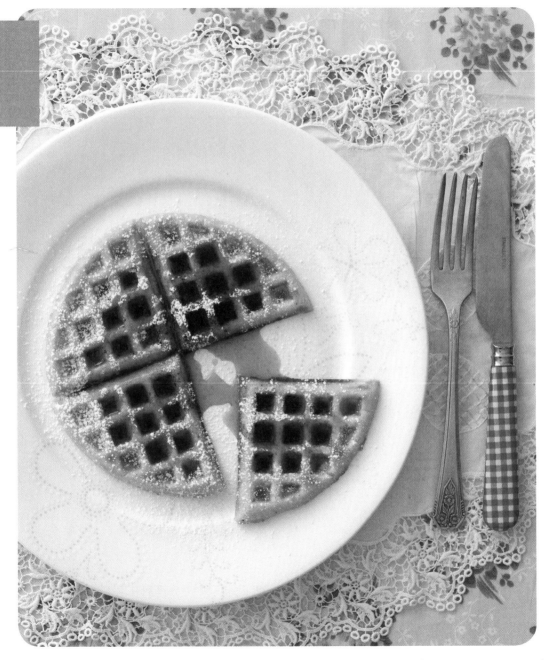

Handy hint Baking powder is a rising agent; it consists of one part baking soda to two parts cream of tartar. Gluten-free baking powder, found in health-food stores, is made without cereal additives.

waffles with maple syrup

This recipe is also gluten-free.

7 oz dairy-free spread
¾ cup superfine sugar
1 teaspoon vanilla extract
3 eggs, separated
1¼ cups potato flour
1 cup brown rice flour
1 teaspoon gluten-free baking powder
1 cup water
cooking oil spray
2 teaspoons confectioners' sugar
1 cup pure maple syrup

1 Beat spread, superfine sugar, and extract in medium bowl with electric mixer until light and fluffy. Beat in egg yolks, one at a time.

2 Beat egg whites in small bowl with electric mixer until soft peaks form; fold into egg yolk mixture.

3 Fold in sifted dry ingredients and water. Do not over-mix (mixture may look slightly curdled).

4 Spray heated waffle iron with cooking spray; pour ½ cup of batter over bottom element of waffle iron. Close iron; cook waffle about 3 minutes or until browned on both sides and crisp. Transfer waffle to plate; cover to keep warm. Repeat with cooking oil and remaining batter to make a total of 12 waffles.

5 Serve waffles dusted with sifted confectioners' sugar and maple syrup.

prep + cook time 45 minutes makes 12 nutritional count per waffle 388 calories; 15.8 g total fat (2.9 g saturated fat); 58.1 g carbohydrate; 0.8 g fiber; 3 g protein

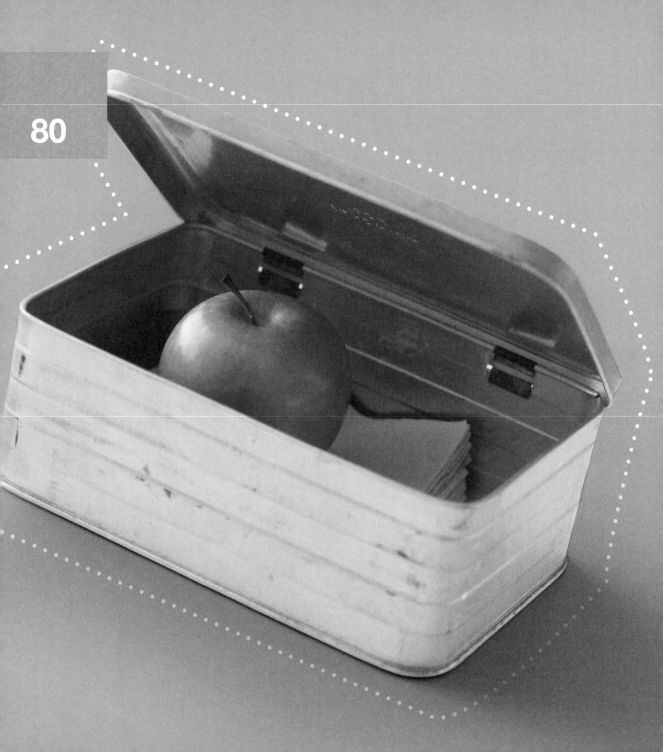

My favorite recipes

....

....

....

....

....

....

....

....

My lunchbox Always pack lunches with a frozen drink or an ice pack to keep them cool and fresh until lunchtime.

rice noodle cakes

This recipe is also nut-free and gluten-free.

7 oz rice vermicelli noodles
1 medium carrot (4 oz), coarsely grated
1 medium zucchini (4 oz), coarsely grated
½ cup coarsely chopped fresh cilantro
3 eggs, beaten lightly
2 tablespoons gluten-free sweet chili sauce
2 tablespoons vegetable oil

1 Place noodles in large heatproof bowl; cover with boiling water. Stand 5 minutes or until tender; drain. Cut noodles coarsely with kitchen scissors.
2 Combine noodles, carrot, zucchini, cilantro, eggs, and sauce in large bowl.
3 Heat a little of the oil in large frying pan over medium heat; cook ¼ cup of mixture, flattening slightly with spatula, until browned on both sides. Repeat with remaining oil and noodle mixture, cooking three or four cakes at a time, to make a total of 20 noodle cakes.

Pack noodle cakes and a dipping sauce in separate containers, in the lunchbox.

prep + cook time 35 minutes makes 20 nutritional count per noodle cake 63 calories; 2.8 g total fat (0.5 g saturated fat); 7.2 g carbohydrate; 0.5 g fiber; 1.8 g protein

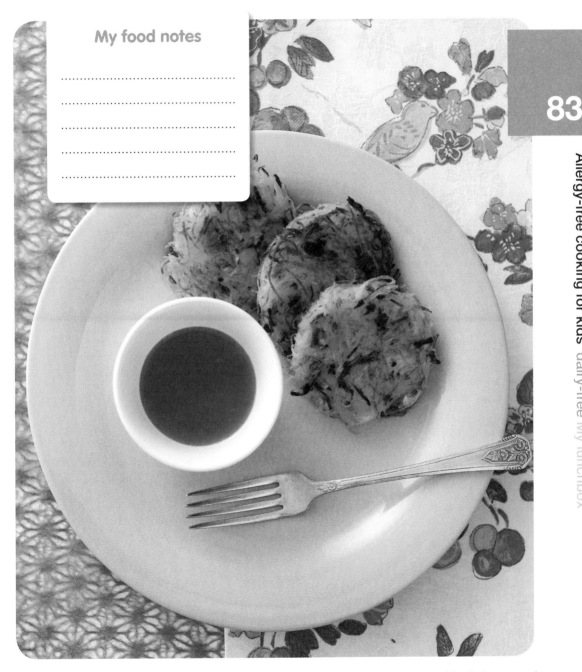

My food notes

....
....
....
....
....

Did you know? Rice vermicelli noodles, used throughout Asia in spring rolls and cold salads, are made with rice flour and are different from bean thread vermicelli, which are made from mung bean starch.

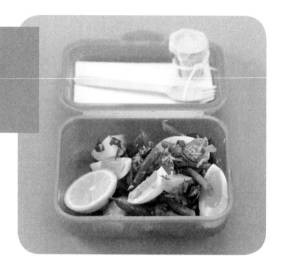

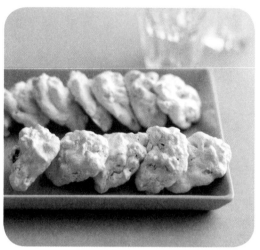

niçoise salad

This recipe is also nut-free and gluten-free.

3½ oz baby new potatoes, quartered
2 oz green beans, halved
3 oz can tuna in spring water, drained
1 hard-boiled egg, quartered
1 tablespoon pitted black olives
1 tablespoons coarsely chopped fresh
flat-leaf parsley

1 Cook potatoes and beans separately, until tender. Rinse; drain.
2 Combine potato and beans with flaked tuna, egg, olives, and parsley in medium bowl. Pack salad with half a lemon.

prep + cook time 10 minutes serves 1
nutritional count per serving 282 calories;
7.8 g total fat (2.4 g saturated fat);
20.3 g carbohydrate; 4.9 g fiber; 29.7 g protein

fruity macaroons

3 egg whites
¾ cup superfine sugar
½ cup desiccated (dried) coconut
2 tablespoons all-purpose flour
2 cups air-popped popcorn
½ cup (3 oz) finely chopped dried apricots

1 Preheat oven to 300°F/275°F convection. Grease baking sheets; line with parchment.
2 Beat egg whites in small bowl with electric mixer until soft peaks form. Add sugar; beat until dissolved. Transfer to large bowl; fold in coconut, sifted flour, then popcorn and apricots.
3 Drop tablespoons of mixture about 2 inches apart onto pans; bake about 20 minutes. Cool on pans.

prep + cook time 35 minutes makes 24
nutritional count per macaroon 54 calories;
1.1 g total fat (1 g saturated fat);
9.5 g carbohydrate; 0.8 g fiber; 0.9 g protein

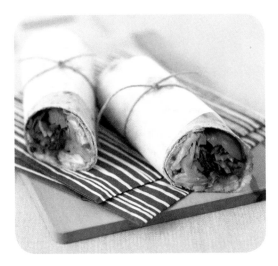

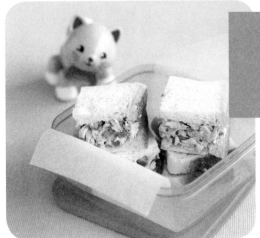

lavash wrap

This recipe is also nut-free and egg-free.

1 piece whole-wheat lavash
¼ small avocado (2 oz)
1 teaspoon tahini (sesame seed paste)
½ cup coarsely grated uncooked red beet
⅓ cup coarsely grated uncooked pumpkin
¼ small red peppers (1 oz), thinly sliced
1½ oz button mushrooms, thinly sliced
¼ small red onion (1 oz), thinly sliced

1 Spread avocado and tahini on bread.
2 Place beets, pumpkin, peppers, mushrooms, and onion on long side of bread; roll to enclose filling. Cut in half, then wrap in parchment.

prep + cook time 15 minutes serves 2
nutritional count per serving 184 calories; 6.7 g total fat (1.3 g saturated fat); 22.3 g carbohydrate; 5 g fiber; 6.1 g protein

chicken sandwich

This recipe is also nut-free and egg-free.

⅓ cup finely shredded cooked chicken
1 stalk celery (5 oz), trimmed, finely chopped
¼ small avocado (2 oz)
1 teaspoon lemon juice
2 slices white sandwich bread

1 Combine chicken, celery, avocado, and juice in small bowl. Sandwich mixture between bread slices; cut as desired. Wrap in parchment or plastic wrap.

preparation time 10 minutes makes 1
nutritional count per sandwich
324 calories; 13.2 g total fat (3 g saturated fat); 30.1 g carbohydrate; 4.2 g fiber; 19 g protein

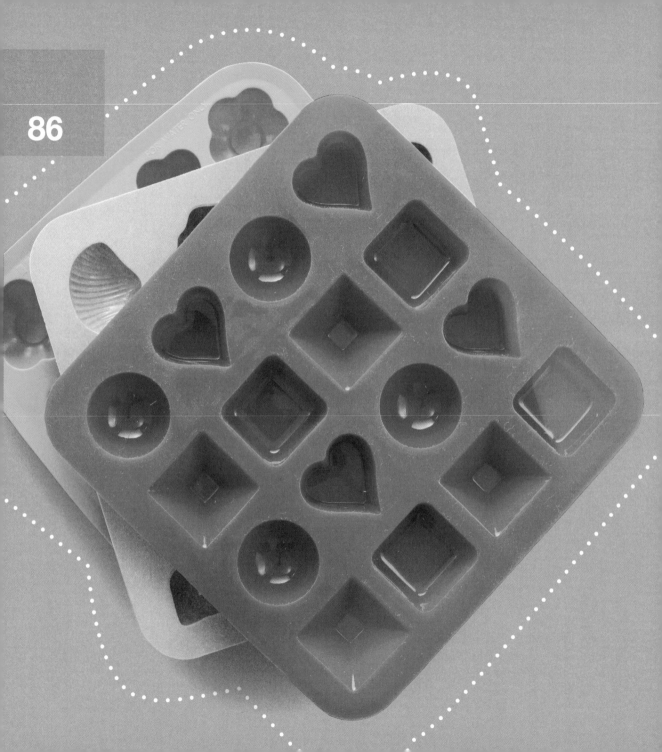

My favorite recipes

....
....
....
....
....
....
....
....
....

After-school snacks Ice pops, chocolate cake, or a rice paper chicken roll—all so yummy you'll definitely want to share.

hoisin and barbecue chicken rolls

This recipe is also nut-free and egg-free.

½ Lebanese cucumber (2 oz)
½ medium carrot (2 oz)
12 7-inch-square rice paper sheets
2 tablespoons hoisin sauce
1¼ cups finely shredded cooked chicken
2 oz snow peas, trimmed, thinly sliced

1 Using vegetable peeler, slice cucumber and carrot into ribbons.
2 To assemble rolls, place one sheet of rice paper in medium bowl of warm water until just softened; lift sheet carefully from water, placing it on a towel-covered board with a corner point facing toward you. Place a little of the sauce and chicken vertically along center of sheet; top with a little of the cucumber, carrot, and snow peas. Fold corner point facing you up over filling; roll rice paper sheet side to side to enclose filling. Repeat with remaining rice paper sheets and filling ingredients.

prep + cook time 20 minutes makes 12 nutritional count per roll 44 calories; 1.1 g total fat (0.3 g saturated fat); 5 g carbohydrate; 0.8 g fiber; 3.1 g protein

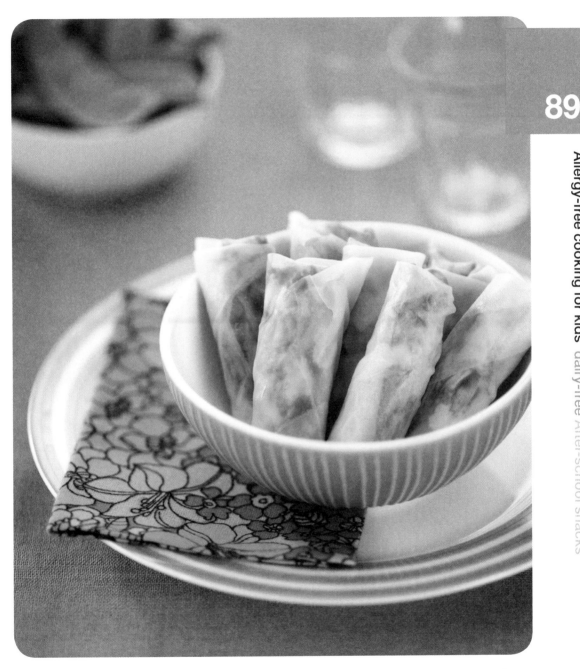

Did you know? Lebanese cucumbers are short, slender, and thin-skinned. They are probably the most popular variety because of their tender, edible skin; tiny, yielding seeds; and sweet, fresh taste.

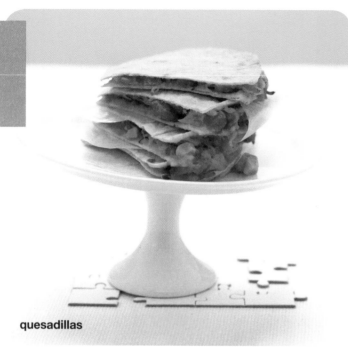

quesadillas

prep + cook time
30 minutes
makes 4
nutritional count
per quesadilla
338 calories;
19.8 g total fat
(2.9 g saturated fat);
22.6 g carbohydrate;
7.8 g fiber;
13.8 g protein

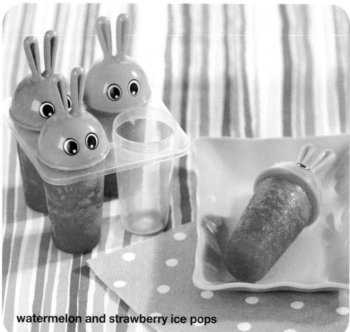

watermelon and strawberry ice pops

prep + cook time
15 minutes
(+ refrigeration and
freezing) makes 4
nutritional count per
ice pop 57 calories;
0.2 g total fat
(0 g saturated fat);
12.7 g carbohydrate;
0.8 g fiber;
0.5 g protein

quesadillas

This recipe is also nut-free and egg-free.

2 medium tomatoes (11 oz), seeded,
   finely chopped
1 medium avocado (9 oz), finely chopped
1 medium zucchini (4 oz), coarsely grated
½ small red onion (2 oz), finely chopped
4 oz can corn kernels, rinsed, drained
15 oz can Mexican-style beans, rinsed,
   drained
1 cup (5 oz) coarsely grated soy cheese
8 small corn tortillas

1 Preheat sandwich press.
2 Combine vegetables and beans in
medium bowl.
3 Divide bean mixture and cheese over
four tortillas, leaving ¾-inch border around
edge; top each with the remaining tortillas.
4 Cook quesadillas, one at a time, in
sandwich press until browned lightly. Cut
into halves or quarters to serve.

watermelon and strawberry ice pops

This recipe is also nut-free, gluten-free,
and egg-free.

⅓ cup water
2 tablespoons white sugar
12 oz watermelon, peeled, seeded,
   coarsely chopped
3 oz strawberries, coarsely chopped
2 teaspoons lemon juice

1 Combine water and sugar in small
saucepan; stir over low heat until sugar
dissolves. Bring to a boil; boil uncovered,
without stirring, about 2 minutes, or until
mixture thickens slightly. Transfer syrup
to small bowl; refrigerate until cold.
2 Blend or process cold syrup with
watermelon, strawberries, and lemon juice
until smooth. Pour mixture into four ⅓-cup
popsicle molds. Freeze until firm, stirring
occasionally during freezing to stop
mixture from separating.

chocolate-on-chocolate cakes

This recipe is also gluten-free.

7 oz dairy-free spread, softened
2¼ cups gluten-free self-rising flour
¼ cup cocoa powder
1 cup superfine sugar
¾ cup gluten-free soy milk
2 eggs
2 egg whites
chocolate icing
1 cup confectioners' sugar
1 tablespoon cocoa powder
2 tablespoons water

1 Preheat oven to 350°F/325°F convection. Line two 12-hole (¹/₃-cup) muffin pans with paper liners.
2 Beat spread in large bowl with electric mixer until pale. Beat sifted flour, cocoa, and ¼ cup of the sugar alternately with milk into spread, in two batches, until combined.
3 Beat eggs and egg whites in small bowl with electric mixer until thick and creamy. Gradually add remaining sugar, one tablespoon at a time, beating until sugar dissolves between additions. Gradually beat egg mixture into flour mixture until combined.
4 Drop 2½ tablespoons mixture into each paper liner; bake cakes about 20 minutes. Turn, top-side up, onto wire rack to cool.
5 Make chocolate icing. Spread chocolate icing on cooled cakes.
chocolate icing Sift sugar and cocoa into small bowl; stir in water.

prep + cook time 40 minutes (+ cooling) makes 24 nutritional count per cake 152 calories; 7.8 g total fat (4.9 g saturated fat); 27.4 g carbohydrate; 0.2 g fiber; 1.6 g protein

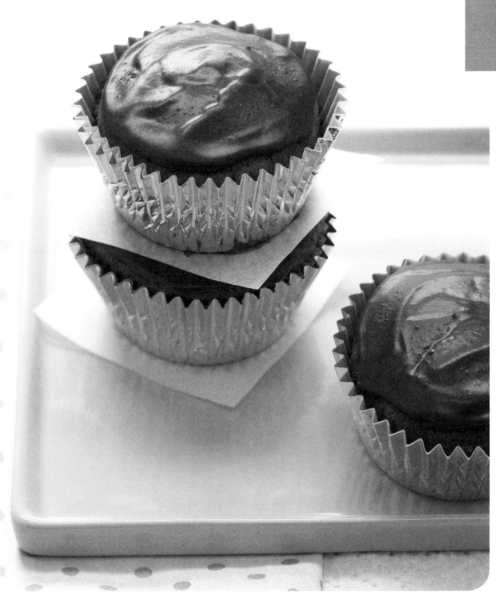

Healthy tip Soy milk is made by soaking soy beans in water, grinding the beans, then filtering the liquid; it has a nutty flavor. It contains iron and vitamins B1 and B3; however, it is low in calcium.

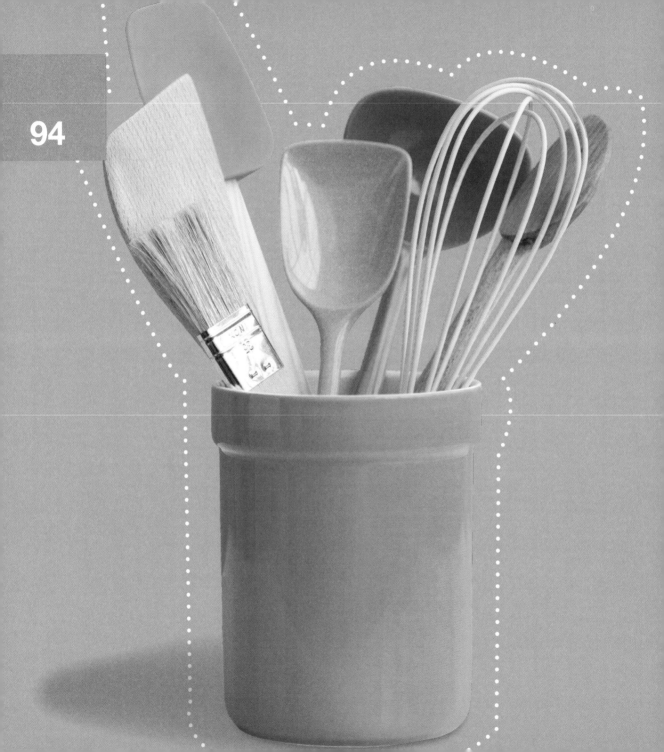

My favorite recipes

....
....
....
....
....
....
....
....
....

These dinner-time meals, cooked with minimum fuss, are sure to become regular family favorites.

chicken noodle soup

3 cups chicken stock

1 quart water

**3 chicken breast filets (21 oz), cut into
⅓-inch strips**

11 oz can corn kernels, drained

2 teaspoons soy sauce

**2 3 oz packets chicken-flavored
ramen noodles**

1 tablespoon chopped fresh chives

1 Combine stock and water in large saucepan, bring to the boil; add chicken, corn, sauce, the chicken-flavor packet from the noodles, and noodles to the pan.

2 Return soup to a boil; reduce heat to medium and cook 5 minutes or until chicken is cooked through.

3 Serve soup garnished with chives.

prep + cook time 15 minutes serves 4 nutritional count per serving 443 calories; 10.3 g total fat (3.1 g saturated fat); 43.5 g carbohydrate; 3.2 g fiber; 41.8 g protein

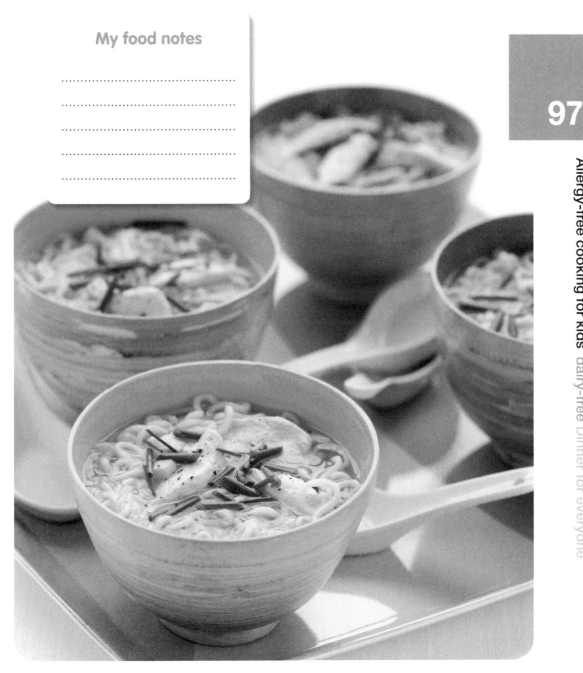

My food notes

....
....
....
....
....

Handy hint Make your own chicken stock by simmering chicken bones, chopped onions, carrots, celery stalks, peppercorns, and bay leaves in 5 quarts of water for about 2 hours; then strain.

chow mein

1 tablespoon vegetable oil
18 oz lean ground beef
1 medium brown onion (5oz),
   finely chopped
2 cloves garlic, crushed
1 tablespoon curry powder
1 large carrot (6 oz), finely chopped
2 stalks celery (11 oz), trimmed,
   thinly sliced
5 oz button mushrooms, thinly sliced
1 cup chicken stock
⅓ cup oyster sauce
2 tablespoons soy sauce
15 oz fresh thin egg noodles
½ cup (2 oz) frozen peas
½ cup (2 oz) frozen sliced green beans
½ small Napa cabbage (14 oz),
   coarsely shredded

1 Heat oil in wok over high heat; stir-fry beef, onion, and garlic until meat is browned. Add curry powder; stir-fry 1 minute or until fragrant. Add carrot and celery; stir-fry until vegetables soften. Add mushrooms, stir-fry until just softened.
2 Add stock, sauces, and noodles to pan, stir-fry gently until combined; bring to a boil. Add peas, beans, and cabbage; simmer, uncovered, tossing occasionally, about 5 minutes, or until vegetables are just soft.

Napa cabbage, also known as wombok, Chinese cabbage, or petsai, is the most common cabbage in Southeast Asian cooking. It is elongated in shape with pale green, crinkly leaves, and is available from Asian grocery stores and most major supermarkets.

prep + cook time 40 minutes serves 4 nutritional count per serving 614 calories; 14.3 g total fat (4.1 g saturated fat); 71.9 g carbohydrate; 8.8 g fiber; 44.1 g protein

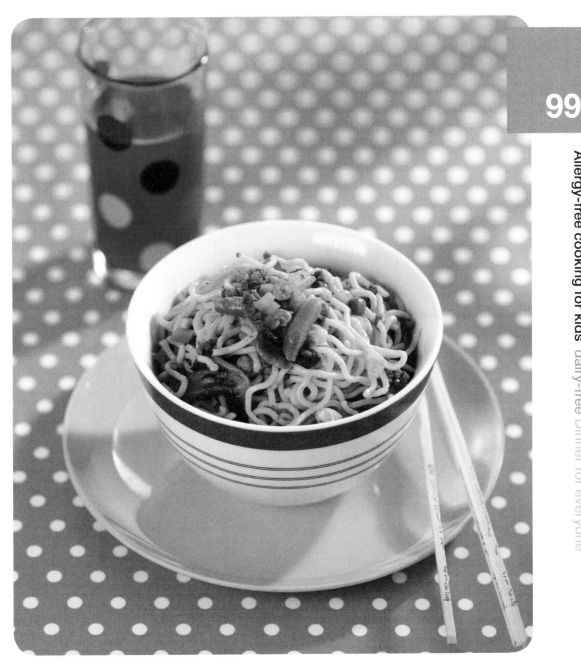

Did you know? In traditional chow mein, the noodles are deep-fried in bundles; this dish is similar to the chao mian of China, which uses softened noodles. Hokkien noodles could also be used.

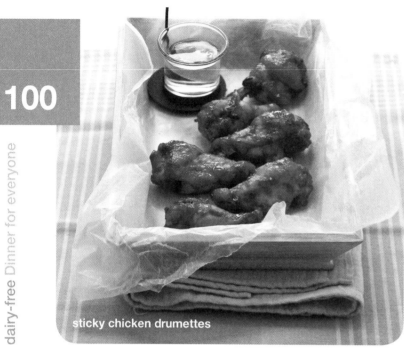

sticky chicken drumettes

prep + cook time
40 minutes
(+ refrigeration)
makes 16
nutritional count
per drumette
91 calories;
3.8 g total fat
(1.1 g saturated fat);
7.8 g carbohydrate;
0.3 g fiber;
6.2 g protein

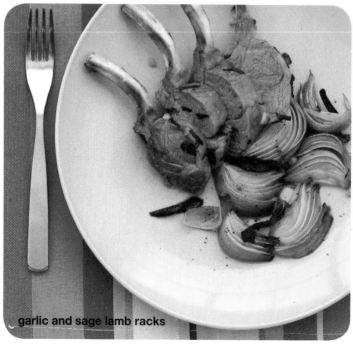

garlic and sage lamb racks

prep + cook time
30 minutes
serves 4
nutritional count
per serving
407 calories;
31.3 g total fat
(8.5 g saturated fat);
12.4 g carbohydrate;
3.4 g fiber;
18.4 g protein

sticky chicken drumettes

This recipe is also nut-free.

¾ cup tomato sauce
⅓ cup plum sauce
2 tablespoons Worcestershire sauce
1 tablespoon brown sugar
16 chicken drumettes (2 lbs)

1 Combine sauces and sugar in large bowl; add chicken. Cover; refrigerate 3 hours or overnight.
2 Preheat oven to 400°F/375°F convection.
3 Drain chicken; discard marinade. Place chicken on oiled wire rack over large baking dish. Roast chicken about 30 minutes, or until cooked through.

Serve with a leafy green salad.

garlic and sage lamb racks

This recipe is also nut-free, gluten-free, and egg-free.

3 large red onions (11 oz)
12 fresh sage leaves
⅓ cup olive oil
2 tablespoons coarsely chopped fresh sage
4 cloves garlic, coarsely chopped
4 4-inch french-trimmed lamb cutlet racks (1⅓ lbs)

1 Preheat oven to 425°F/400°F convection.
2 Halve onions lengthwise, slice into thin wedges; place in large baking dish with sage leaves and half of the oil.
3 Combine remaining oil in small bowl with sage and garlic. Press sage mixture all over lamb; arrange on onions in dish.
4 Roast, uncovered, about 25 minutes, or until lamb is browned all over and cooked as desired. Cover lamb racks; stand 10 minutes before serving.

Serve with a salad or vegetables of your choice.

macaroni and cheese with peas

This recipe is also nut-free and gluten-free.

8 oz packet gluten-free spiral pasta
2 tablespoons dairy-free spread
2 tablespoons (100% corn) cornstarch
1½ cups water
1 cup gluten-free soy milk
½ cup (2 oz) coarsely grated soy cheese
1 cup (4 oz) frozen baby peas
½ cup stale gluten-free breadcrumbs

1 Preheat oven to 400°F/375°F convection.
2 Cook pasta in large saucepan of boiling water until tender; drain.
3 Meanwhile, melt spread in large saucepan over medium heat, stir in cornstarch; cook, stirring, 1 minute. Gradually add the combined water and milk, stirring constantly, until mixture boils and thickens slightly. Remove from heat; stir in cheese, peas, and pasta.
4 Pour mixture into oiled shallow 1½-quart ovenproof dish; top with breadcrumbs. Bake about 25 minutes, or until browned lightly. Cool before serving.

prep + cook time 50 minutes serves 6 nutritional count per serving 287 calories; 10.4 g total fat (1.4 g saturated fat); 35.1 g carbohydrate; 5.5 g fiber; 10.1 g protein

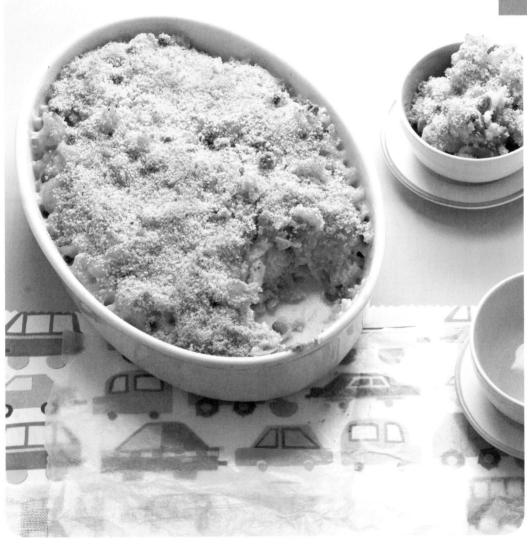

Handy hint If you don't suffer from a gluten allergy, plain breadcrumbs can be used. Make your own breadcrumbs by blending or processing one- or two-day old bread; whole-wheat or white can be used.

My favorite recipes

....

....

....

....

....

....

....

....

....

Seriously sweet Crème brûlée, sticky date cakes, meringue tarts—being on a dairy-free diet never tasted so good.

coconut rice puddings

This recipe is also gluten-free.

4 eggs
⅓ cup superfine sugar
1 teaspoon vanilla extract
13½ oz can coconut cream
1½ cups gluten-free soy milk
1 cup cooked white medium-grain rice
   (see handy hint, page 107)
½ cup golden raisins
½ teaspoon ground cinnamon

1 Preheat oven to 350°F/325°F convection. Grease six ¾-cup ovenproof dishes.
2 Whisk eggs, sugar, and extract in large bowl until combined; whisk in coconut cream and milk. Stir in rice and raisins. Divide mixture evenly among dishes; place dishes in large baking dish. Add enough boiling water to come halfway up sides of small dishes.
3 Bake puddings 20 minutes, whisking gently with fork under the skin of the puddings twice—this stops the rice from sinking to the bottom of the dishes. Sprinkle cinnamon on the puddings; bake a further 20 minutes, or until set. Stand puddings 10 minutes before serving.

prep + cook time 1 hour makes 6 nutritional count per pudding 366 calories; 19.7 g total fat (13.4 g saturated fat); 37.2 g carbohydrate; 2.3 g fiber; 9.1 g protein

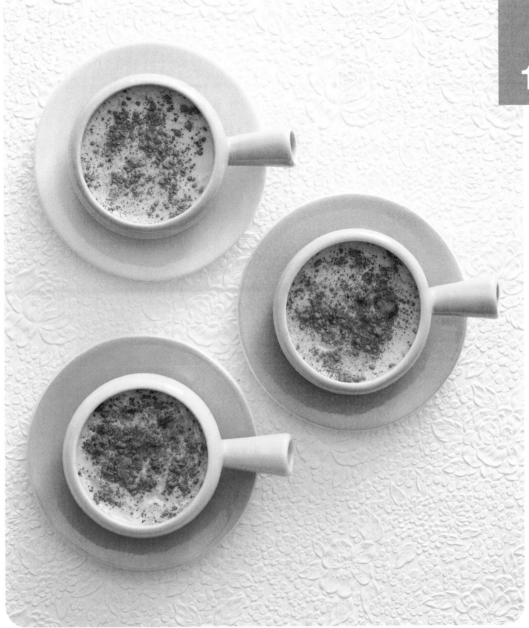

Handy hint You need to cook ⅓ cup white medium-grain rice for this recipe, or you can substitute short-grain rice.

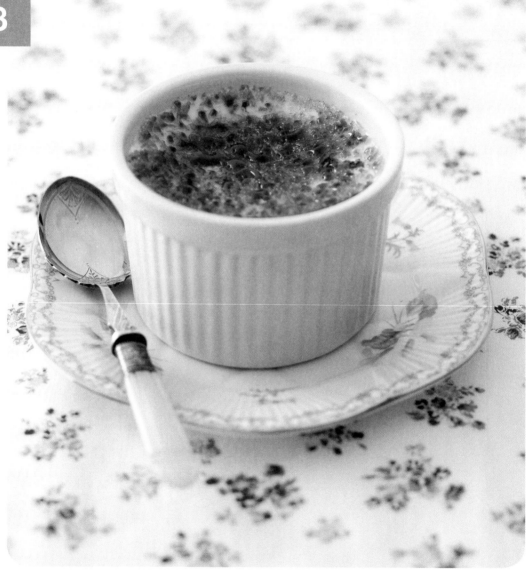

Handy hint Placing the custards in a dish filled with ice cubes keeps them from melting while the sugar is caramelizing under the broiler. Of course, if you have a cooking blowtorch, use that instead.

passionfruit crème brûlée

This recipe is also nut-free and gluten-free.

¼ cup passionfruit pulp
2 egg yolks
1 egg
2 tablespoons superfine sugar
1 teaspoon finely grated lime rind
9 oz can coconut cream
½ cup gluten-free soy milk
1 tablespoon brown sugar

1 Preheat oven to 350°F/325°F convection.

2 Combine passionfruit, egg yolks, egg, sugar, and rind in medium heatproof bowl.

3 Bring coconut cream and milk to a boil in small saucepan. Gradually whisk hot cream mixture into egg mixture. Place bowl over medium saucepan of simmering water; stir over heat about 10 minutes or until custard thickens slightly.

4 Divide custard among four deep ½-cup heatproof dishes. Place dishes in medium baking dish; pour enough boiling water into baking dish to come halfway up sides of small dishes. Bake about 40 minutes or until custard is set. Remove custards from water, cool. Cover, then refrigerate 3 hours or overnight.

5 Preheat broiler.

6 Place custards in shallow flameproof dish filled with ice cubes. Sprinkle each custard with 1 teaspoon brown sugar; using finger, gently smooth sugar over the surface of each custard. Place dish under broiler until sugar caramelizes.

prep + cook time 1 hour (+ cooling and refrigeration) serves 4 nutritional count per serving
269 calories; 19.4 g total fat (14.1 g saturated fat); 16.6 g carbohydrate; 3.5 g fiber; 5.9 g protein

sticky date cakes with orange caramel sauce

This recipe is also gluten-free.

1 cup (5 oz) pitted dried dates
¾ cup boiling water
1 teaspoon baking soda
4 oz dairy-free spread
¾ cup firmly-packed brown sugar
4 eggs
2 cups (8 oz) ground almonds
½ cup desiccated (dried) coconut
½ cup rice flour

orange caramel sauce
3 tablespoons dairy-free spread
½ cup firmly-packed brown sugar
⅓ cup orange juice

1 Preheat oven to 350°F/325°F convection. Grease two 6-hole (¾-cup) jumbo muffin pans; line base of each pan hole with parchment.

2 Combine dates, water, and soda in bowl of food processor. Place lid in position; let stand 5 minutes, then process until almost smooth.

3 Beat spread and sugar in small bowl with electric mixer until light and fluffy. Beat in eggs, one at a time (mixture will curdle). Transfer to large bowl; stir in ground almonds, coconut, and sifted flour, then the date mixture. Divide mixture among pan holes.

4 Bake cakes about 25 minutes. Stand in pan 5 minutes before serving.

5 Make orange caramel sauce.

6 Serve warm cakes with hot orange caramel sauce.

orange caramel sauce Melt spread in small frying pan over low heat. Add sugar; stir until dissolved. Add juice; cook, stirring, until sauce thickens slightly.

prep + cook time 50 minutes makes 12 nutritional count per cake 400 calories; 23.5 g total fat (4.7 g saturated fat); 38.5 g carbohydrate; 3.6 g fiber; 7.3 g protein

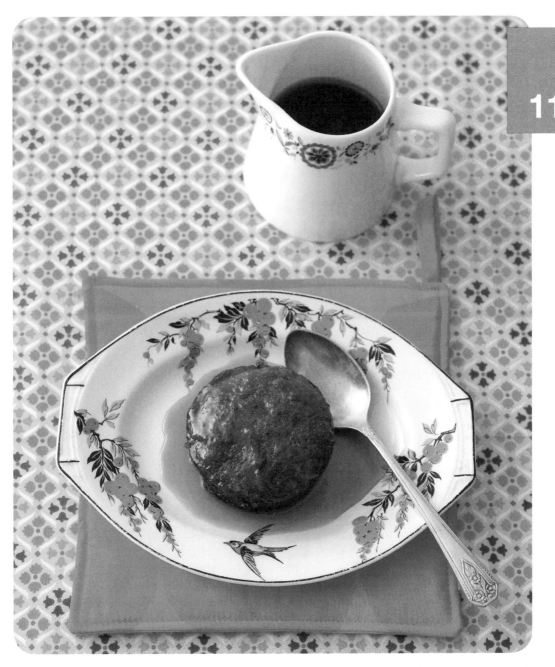

Handy hints An easy way to line the bases of the muffin pan holes is to cut the bottom out of jumbo muffin paper liners and use them. You can substitute ground hazelnuts for the ground almonds.

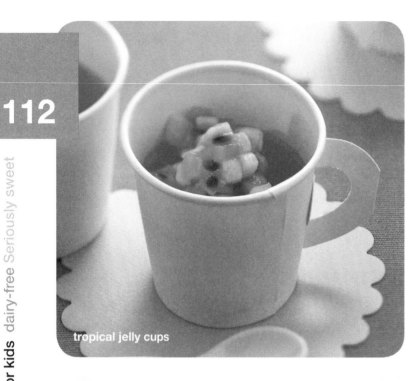

tropical jelly cups

prep + cook time
20 minutes
(+ refrigeration)
makes 12
nutritional count
per jelly cup
48 calories;
0.2 g total fat
(0 g saturated fat);
9.5 g carbohydrate;
1.1 g fiber;
1.4 g protein

berry granola baked apples

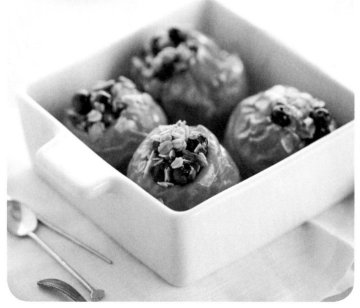

prep + cook time
1 hour 10 minutes
serves 4
nutritional count
per serving
163 calories;
5.4 g total fat
(2.9 g saturated fat);
26 g carbohydrate;
4.4 g fiber;
1.4 g protein

tropical jelly cups

This recipe is also nut-free, egg-free, and gluten-free.

1 tablespoon powdered gelatin
¼ cup water
2¾ cups tropical fruit juice
tropical salsa
1 medium banana (7 oz), finely chopped
½ medium mango (7 oz), finely chopped
¼ cup passionfruit pulp

1 Sprinkle gelatin over the water in small heatproof bowl; stand in small saucepan of simmering water, stirring, until gelatin dissolves.
2 Combine juice and gelatin mixture in large pitcher; pour ¼ cup mixture into twelve ½-cup serving cups. Cover, refrigerate 3 hours or until set.
3 Make tropical salsa.
4 Just before serving, spoon level tablespoons of salsa into each cup.
tropical salsa Combine ingredients in a small bowl.

berry granola baked apples

This recipe is also egg-free.

4 large granny smith apples (1¾ lbs)
cooking oil spray
⅓ cup natural granola
½ cup fresh blueberries
1 tablespoon dairy-free spread, melted
3 teaspoons brown sugar

1 Preheat oven to 325°F/300°F convection.
2 Core unpeeled apples about three-quarters of the way down from stem end, making hole 1½ inches in diameter. Use small sharp knife to score around center of each apple; lightly spray with cooking oil.
3 Combine remaining ingredients in small bowl. Divide mixture among apples, pressing firmly into holes; place apples in small baking dish. Bake, uncovered, about 45 minutes, or until apples are just softened.

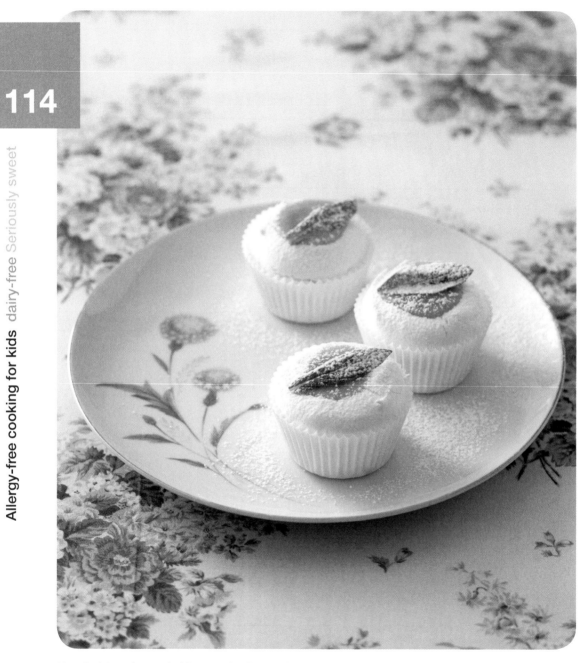

Handy hints Instead of lime, make the curd using lemon, or even orange juice. Make double the curd mixture and use it to fill mini pastry tartlet shells, or use it as a topping for scones or biscuits.

lime curd meringue tarts

This recipe is also nut-free and gluten-free.

2 egg whites
½ cup superfine sugar
2 teaspoons confectioners' sugar
6 fresh mint leaves
1 teaspoon confectioners' sugar, extra
lime curd
2 eggs, beaten lightly
½ cup superfine sugar
3 oz dairy-free spread
⅓ cup lime juice
2 teaspoons finely grated lime rind
green food coloring

1 Preheat oven to 250°F/225°F convection. Line 6-hole (⅓-cup) muffin pan with paper liners.

2 Beat egg whites in small bowl with electric mixer until soft peaks form; gradually add sugars, one tablespoon at a time, beating until sugar dissolves between additions.

3 Spoon meringue into paper liners; using the back of a metal spoon, make a small hollow in each meringue.

4 Bake meringues about 1 hour; cool in oven with door ajar.

5 Meanwhile, make lime curd.

6 Serve meringues topped with curd, then mint leaves. Dust with extra sifted confectioners' sugar.

lime curd Strain eggs into medium heatproof bowl, stir in sugar, spread, and juice; stir over medium saucepan of simmering water until mixture thickens and coats the back of a wooden spoon. Remove from heat. Stand bowl in sink of cold water, stirring occasionally, about 10 minutes or until cold. Stir in rind and tint with food coloring. Cover; refrigerate 1 hour or until thick.

prep + cook time 1 hour 15 minutes (+ cooling and refrigeration) makes 6 nutritional count per meringue 293 calories; 13.9 g total fat (2.7 g saturated fat); 38.4 g carbohydrate; 0.9 g fiber; 3.6 g protein

chocolate hazelnut cake

This recipe is also gluten-free.

3½ oz dairy-free spread
½ cup firmly packed brown sugar
2 eggs
¼ cup gluten-free soy milk
¾ cup (3 oz) ground hazelnuts
¾ cup gluten-free self-rising flour
2 tablespoons cocoa powder
fudge frosting
3 tablespoons dairy-free spread
¼ cup superfine sugar
2 tablespoons water
¾ cup confectioners' sugar
2 tablespoons cocoa powder

1 Preheat oven to 350°F/325°F convection. Grease shallow 9-inch-square cake pan; line base and sides with parchment, extending paper 2 inches over sides.

2 Beat spread and sugar in medium bowl with electric mixer until changed to a paler color. Beat in eggs, one at a time. Stir in milk, ground nuts, sifted flour, and cocoa, in two batches.

3 Spread mixture into pan; bake about 20 minutes. Stand cake in pan 10 minutes before inverting onto wire rack to cool.

4 Meanwhile, make fudge frosting. Spread frosting over cooled cake.

fudge frosting Combine spread, sugar, and water in small saucepan; stir over low heat until sugar dissolves. Transfer to medium bowl; gradually stir in sifted confectioners' sugar and cocoa until smooth. Cover; refrigerate 20 minutes. Beat frosting with electric mixer until spreadable.

prep + cook time 40 minutes serves 25 nutritional count per serving 122 calories; 7.4 g total fat (1.2 g saturated fat); 15.3 g carbohydrate; 0.4 g fiber; 1.4 g protein

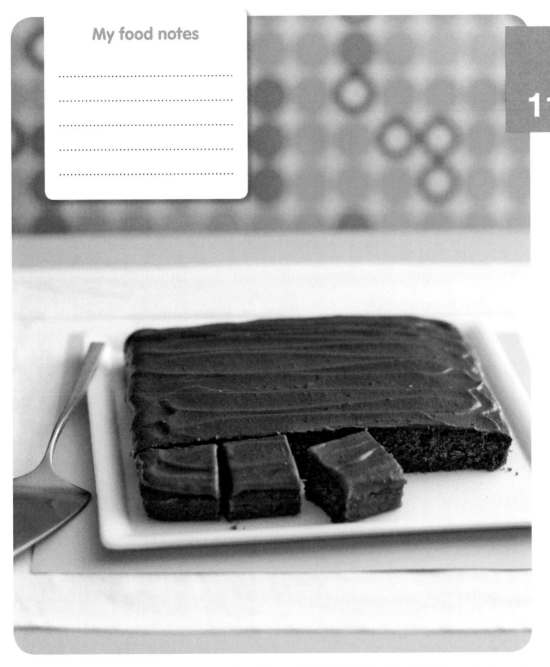

My food notes

....
....
....
....
....

Handy hint This delicious fudgy cake is gluten-free, so it's just the thing for a birthday party. Decorate the top using the many gluten-free cake decorations available from the cake decorating stores or online.

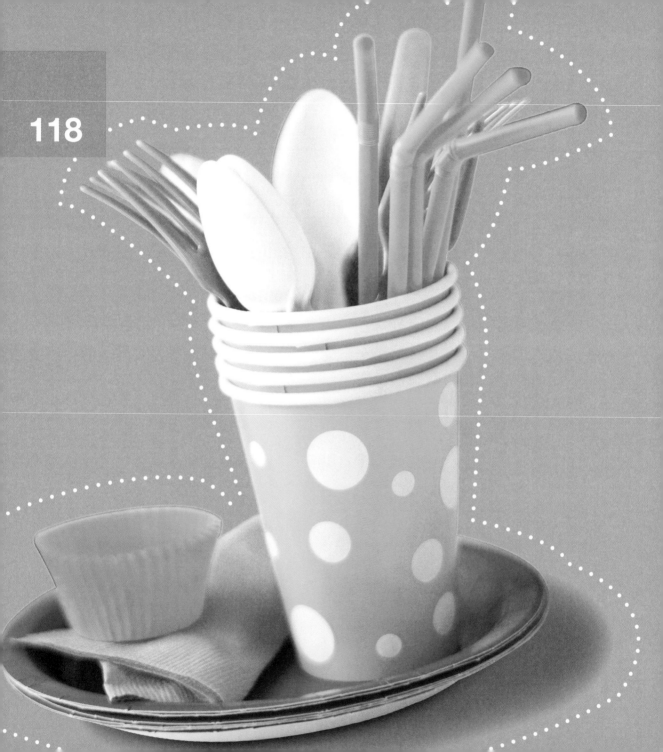

My favorite recipes

....
....
....
....
....
....
....
....
....

Party time Not just for those on a "special" diet, these recipes will have everyone heading back to the table for more treats.

veggie rice paper rolls

This recipe is also nut-free, gluten-free, and egg-free.

1 large carrot (6 oz), coarsely grated
2 stalks celery (10½ oz), trimmed,
  finely chopped
5 oz Napa cabbage, finely shredded
½ cup bean sprouts, coarsely chopped
2 tablespoons lemon juice
1 tablespoon fish sauce
2 teaspoons brown sugar
24 7-inch-square rice paper sheets
24 fresh mint leaves

1 Combine carrot, celery, cabbage, sprouts, juice, sauce, and sugar in medium bowl.

2 Place one sheet of rice paper in medium bowl of warm water until just softened. Lift sheet from water carefully; place on a towel-covered board with a corner pointing toward you.

3 Place 1 rounded tablespoon of vegetable mixture horizontally in center of sheet; top with one mint leaf. Fold corner facing you over filling; roll to cover filling, then fold in sides. Continue rolling to enclose filling. Repeat with remaining rice paper sheets, vegetable mixture, and mint leaves.

prep time 35 minutes makes 24 nutritional count per roll 23 calories; 0.2 g total fat (0 g saturated fat); 4 g carbohydrate; 0.7 g fiber; 0.9 g protein

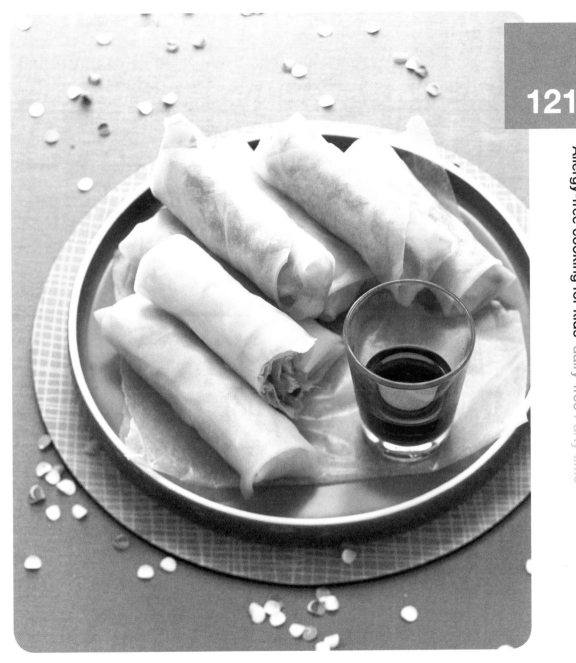

Handy hint For a twist, add softened rice vermicelli noodles and cooked chicken tenderloin. Serve with gluten-free tamari (soy) sauce or sweet chili sauce.

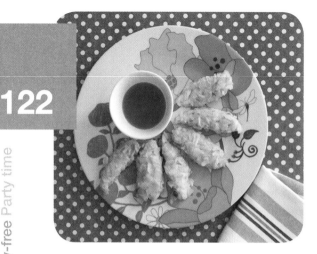

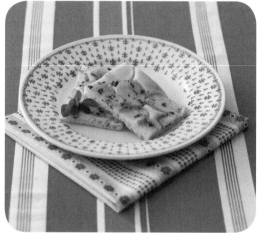

chicken fingers

This recipe is also gluten-free.

8 chicken tenderloins (1⅓ lbs)
3½ oz packet gluten-free potato chips
1 egg white
⅓ cup gluten-free sweet chili sauce

1 Preheat oven to 400°F/375°F convection.
2 Cut tenderloins in half diagonally.
3 Coarsely crush chips; place in medium shallow bowl. Whisk egg white lightly in small shallow bowl.
4 Dip chicken in egg white, then in chips to coat; place, in single layer, on oiled wire rack over baking sheet. Bake about 15 minutes, or until chicken is cooked through. Serve fingers with sauce.

prep + cook time 30 minutes makes 16
nutritional count per finger 90 calories;
4.2 g total fat (1.5 g saturated fat);
4 g carbohydrate; 1 g fiber; 8.7 g protein

potato pizza

This recipe is also gluten-free.

13 oz packet gluten-free bread mix
10½ oz baby new potatoes, thinly sliced
2 teaspoons chopped fresh oregano
2 teaspoons olive oil
1 clove garlic, crushed

1 Preheat oven to 425°F/400°F convection. Oil two 9 x 13-inch jelly roll pans; line bases with parchment, extending paper 2 inches over long sides.
2 Make bread mix according to packet directions; spread mixture into pans.
3 Combine remaining ingredients in medium bowl; spread potato mixture over bread mix.
4 Bake 20 minutes or until potato is tender and crusts are crisp.

prep + cook time 45 minutes serves 6
nutritional count per serving 267 calories;
2.3 g total fat (0.4 g saturated fat); 40.9 g
carbohydrate; 2.8 g fiber; 8.1 g protein

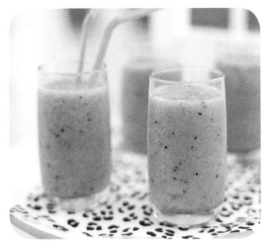

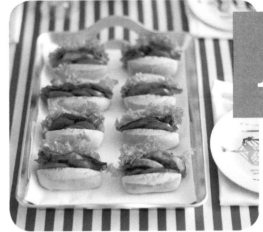

kiwi slushy

This recipe is also nut-free.

12 kiwi
3½ cups ice cubes
3 cups chilled kiwi mix fruit juice

1 Peel kiwi, quarter lengthwise; remove core and as many black seeds as possible.
2 Just before serving, blend kiwi, ice cubes, and juice, in batches, until almost smooth. Pour slush into large pitcher to serve.

prep + cook time 20 minutes serves 12
nutritional count per serving 68 calories;
0.2 g total fat (0 g saturated fat); 13.6 g carbohydrate; 2.9 g fiber; 1.4 g protein

baby BLTs

12 "bake at home" dinner rolls
6 bacon strips
⅓ cup dairy-free mayonnaise
12 green leaf lettuce leaves
2 small tomatoes (6 oz), thinly sliced

1 Preheat oven to 350°F/325°F convection.
2 Bake bread rolls 5 minutes. Split in half almost all the way through.
3 Cut bacon in half crosswise; cook bacon in heated large frying pan over medium heat until crisp. Drain on paper towels.
4 Spread mayonnaise inside rolls; fill rolls with lettuce, bacon, and tomato.

prep + cook time 30 minutes serves 12
nutritional count per serving 215 calories;
8.6 g total fat (2.1 g saturated fat);
23.3 g carbohydrate; 1.9 g fiber; 10.2 g protein

chicken spring rolls

This recipe is also nut-free.

2 cups water
1 chicken breast filet (7 oz)
1 medium carrot (4 oz), coarsely grated
½ cup bean sprouts, finely chopped
1 tablespoon finely chopped
    fresh cilantro
1 tablespoon light soy sauce
50 wonton wrappers (see handy hint,
    page 125)

1 Bring the water to a boil in small saucepan; add chicken. Reduce heat; simmer, covered, 10 minutes or until chicken is cooked through. Cool chicken in poaching liquid 10 minutes; drain, finely shred chicken using two forks.
2 Preheat oven to 425°F/400°F convection. Grease and line baking sheet with parchment.
3 Combine chicken, carrot, sprouts, cilantro, and sauce in medium bowl.
4 Place rounded teaspoons of chicken mixture along bottom edge of each wrapper. Fold in sides then moisten top edge with water; roll to enclose filling. Place on tray.
5 Bake about 15 minutes or until rolls are browned lightly and crisp.

prep + cook time 45 minutes makes 50 nutritional count per roll 12 calories; 0.3 g total fat (0 g saturated fat); 0.3 g carbohydrate; 0 g fiber; 1.8 g protein

....
....
....
....
....

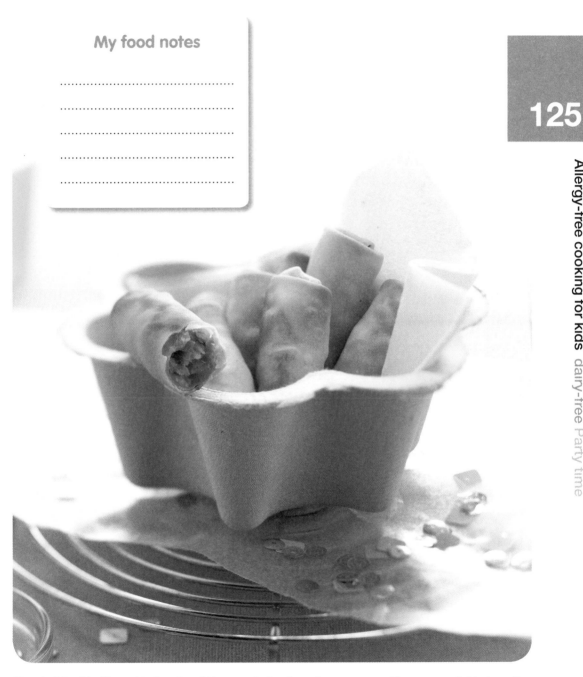

Handy hint You'll need to buy two 9½ oz packets of wonton wrappers. They are available from the refrigerated section of Asian grocery stores and most major supermarkets.

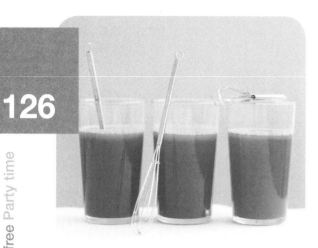

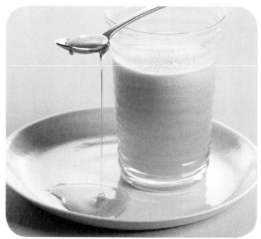

watermelon raspberry juice

This recipe is also nut-free and egg-free.

4 lbs watermelon
2 cups chilled lemonade
¼ cup non-alcoholic raspberry syrup

1 Remove skin and seeds from melon; coarsely chop flesh. Push flesh through juice extractor, blend, or process, in batches, until mushy.
2 Strain juice into large pitcher; stir in lemonade and syrup.

prep time 10 minutes serves 6
nutritional count per serving 122 calories;
0.7 g total fat (0 g saturated fat);
26.6 g carbohydrate; 2 g fiber; 1 g protein

pineapple and orange juice

This recipe is also nut-free, gluten-free, and egg-free.

1 medium pineapple (2 lbs), peeled,
  coarsely chopped
6 medium oranges (3 lbs), peeled, quartered
1 tablespoon honey

1 Push fruit through juice extractor into glass. Add honey; stir to combine.

prep time 5 minutes serves 4
nutritional count per serving 195 calories;
0.4 g total fat (0 g saturated fat);
38.5 g carbohydrate; 8.5 g fiber; 4.5 g protein

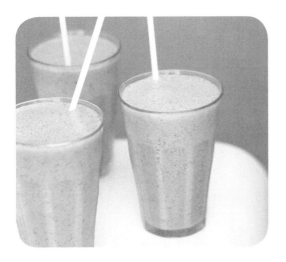

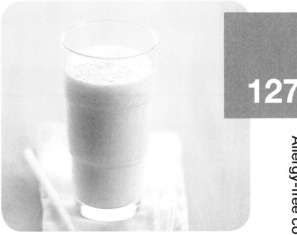

mixed berry soy smoothie

This recipe is also gluten-free.

8 oz soy strawberry ice cream,
   slightly softened
1⅓ cups (7 oz) frozen mixed berries
3 cups gluten-free soy milk

1 Blend ingredients, in batches, until mixture is smooth.

prep time 5 minutes serves 4
nutritional count per serving 205 calories;
9.3 g total fat (3.3 g saturated fat);
21 g carbohydrate; 2.9 g fiber; 8.1 g protein

pear soy smoothie

This recipe is also nut-free, gluten-free, and egg-free.

2 medium pears (1 lb), coarsely chopped
2 cups gluten-free soy milk
1 tablespoon honey

1 Blend or process ingredients until mixture is smooth.

prep time 5 minutes serves 4
nutritional count per serving 141 calories;
2.8 g total fat (0 g saturated fat);
25.5 g carbohydrate; 2.6 g fiber; 1.9 g protein

egg-free

Egg substitutes and egg-free custard and cake mixes are now available in health-food stores.

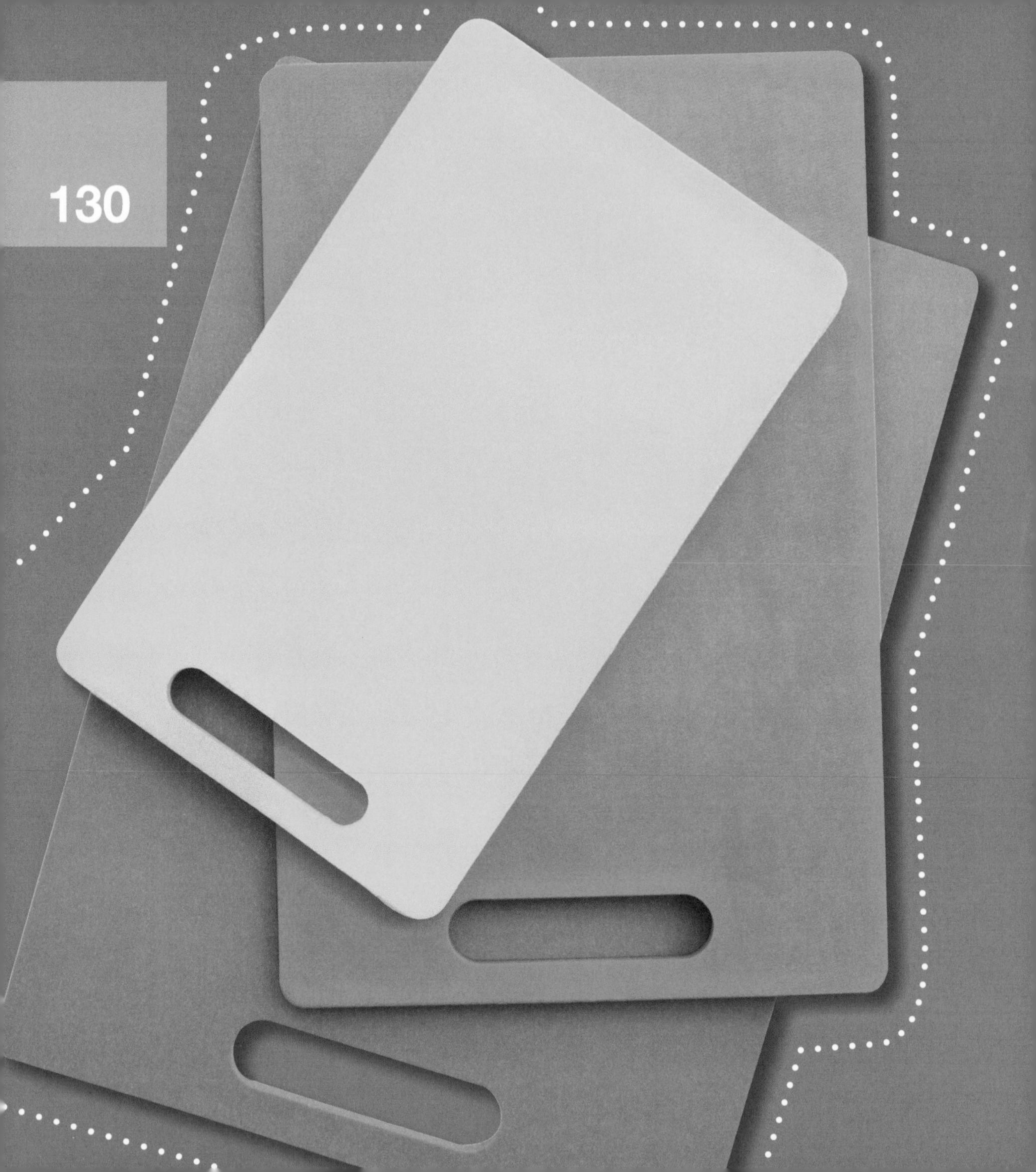

My favorite recipes

....

....

....

....

....

....

....

....

Breakfast Breakfast can lift your mood and has been shown to improve your concentration, which is good for coping at school.

rolled rice porridge

This recipe is also gluten-free and dairy-free.

1½ cups rolled rice
4½ cups water
⅓ cup rice milk
⅓ cup (2 oz) coarsely chopped
  dried apricots
¼ cup flaked coconut, toasted
2 tablespoons honey

1 Combine rolled rice and 3 cups of the water in medium bowl. Cover; stand at room temperature overnight.

2 Place undrained rolled rice in medium saucepan; cook, stirring, until mixture comes to the boil. Add the remaining water; bring to the boil. Reduce heat; simmer, uncovered, about 5 minutes, or until thickened.

3 Divide porridge and milk between serving bowls. Sprinkle apricots and coconut over each; drizzle with honey.

prep + cook time 20 minutes (+ standing) serves 4 nutritional count per serving 252 calories; 2.8 g total fat (1.7 g saturated fat); 50.7 g carbohydrate; 2.7 g fiber; 3.9g protein

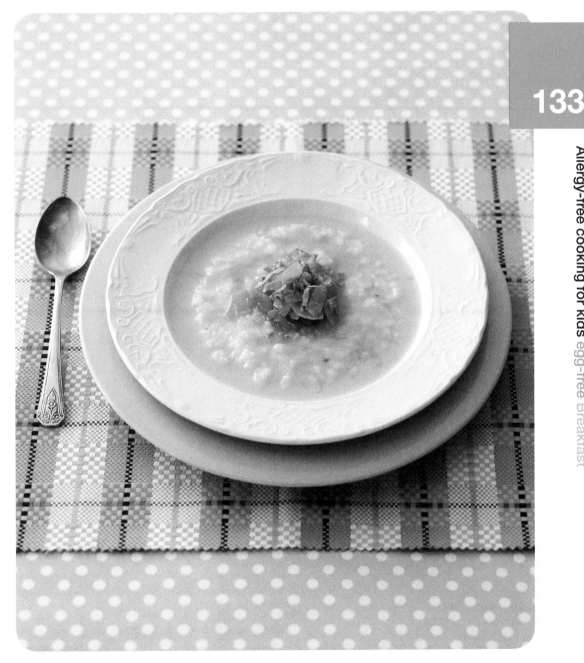

Handy hints You can substitute soy, whole, or skim milk for the rice milk. Instead of the dried apricots, add your favorite chopped dried fruit. Stewed fruit or canned fruit would also work well.

Allergy-free cooking for kids egg-free Breakfast

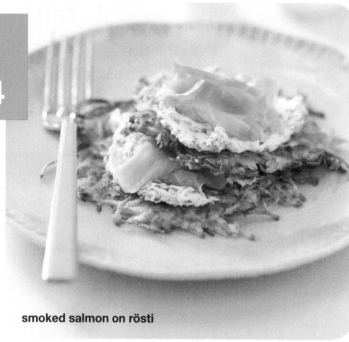

smoked salmon on rösti

prep + cook time
40 minutes
serves 4
nutritional count
per serving
304 calories;
16.1 g total fat
(4.8 g saturated fat);
23.4 g carbohydrate;
2.8 g fiber;
15.3 g protein

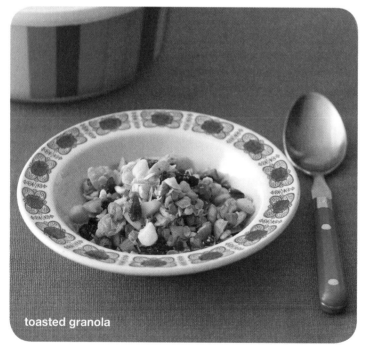

toasted granola

prep + cook time
25 minutes
(+ cooling)
makes 8 cups or
serves 24
(⅓-cup serving)
nutritional count
per ⅓ cup serving
194 calories;
2.7 g total fat
(2.1 g saturated fat);
13.5 g carbohydrate;
2.7 g fiber;
3.7 g protein

smoked salmon on rösti

This recipe is also nut-free and gluten-free.

4 medium potatoes (1¾ lbs), peeled
2 tablespoons vegetable oil
½ cup spreadable
  light cream cheese
1 tablespoon finely chopped fresh
  flat-leaf parsley
1 tablespoon finely chopped fresh chives
1 tablespoon lemon juice
5 oz sliced smoked salmon

1 To make rösti, coarsely grate potatoes; use hands to squeeze out as much excess liquid as possible. Measure ¼ cups of grated potato, placing each portion on a sheet of parchment.
2 Heat 2 teaspoons of oil in large frying pan over medium heat; place two portions of the grated potato in pan, flattening each with spatula. Cook rösti until browned; turn with spatula to cook other side. Drain rösti on paper towels; make six more rösti with remaining oil and grated potato.
3 Combine cream cheese, herbs, and juice in small bowl.
4 Divide rösti between four serving plates; top with herbed cream cheese and smoked salmon.

toasted granola

This recipe is also gluten-free.

2 tablespoons golden syrup or honey
2 tablespoons macadamia or
  vegetable oil
1 cup gluten-free cornflakes
1 cup (5 oz) coarsely chopped macadamias
1 cup (5 oz) coarsely chopped pistachios
1 cup (6 oz) coarsely chopped almonds
1 cup rolled rice
1 cup puffed rice
½ cup flaked coconut
½ cup (3½ oz) finely chopped dried figs
½ cup (2 oz) dried cranberries

1 Preheat oven to 350°F/325°F convection.
2 Combine syrup and oil in small bowl.
3 Combine cornflakes, nuts, rolled rice, puffed rice, and coconut in shallow baking dish; drizzle syrup mixture over it. Roast, uncovered, about 15 minutes, or until browned lightly, stirring halfway through roasting time. Cool 10 minutes.
4 Stir fruit into granola mixture; cool.

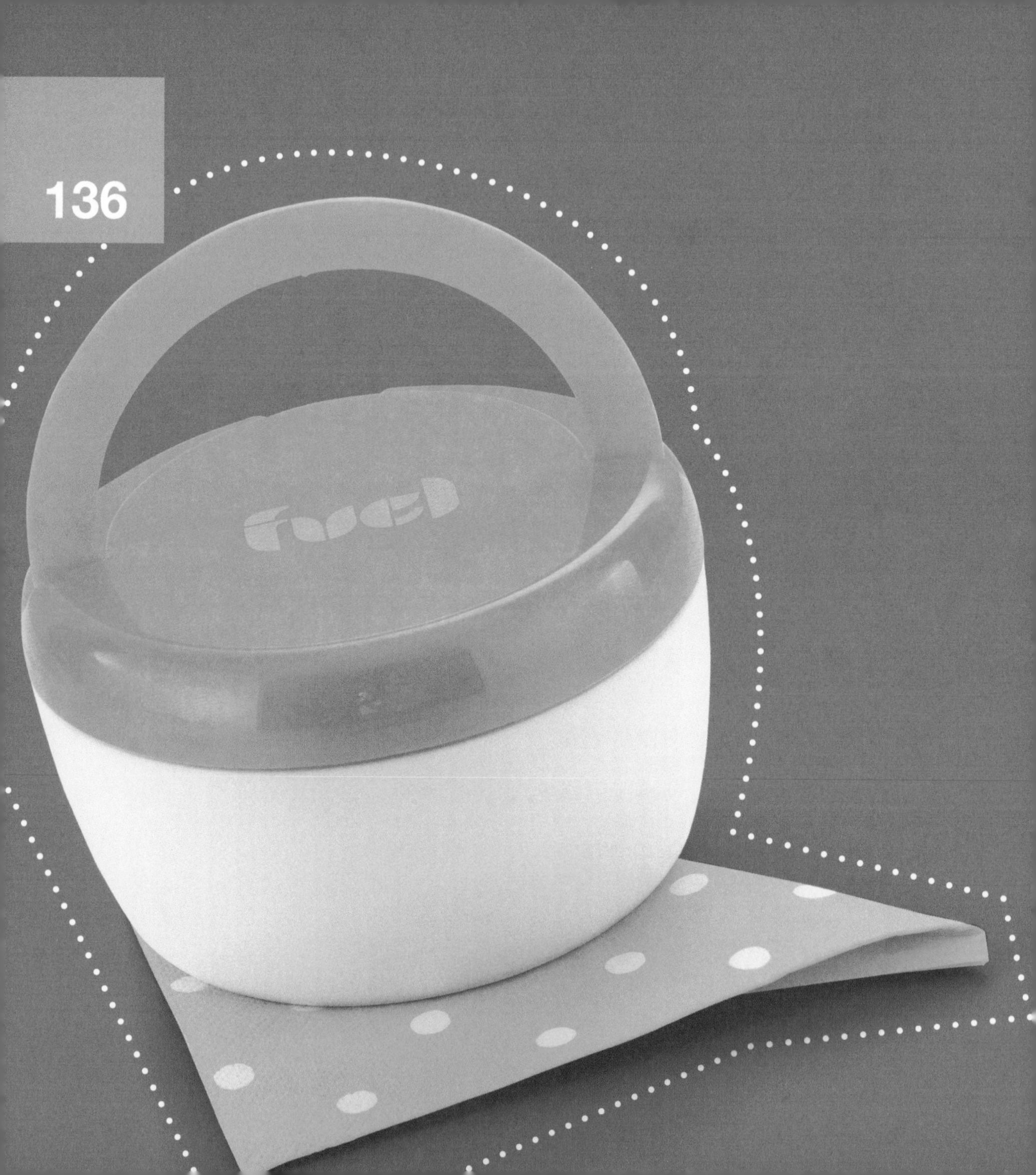

My favorite recipes

....

....

....

....

....

....

....

....

My lunchbox Always pack lunches with a frozen drink or an ice pack to keep them cool and fresh until lunchtime.

zucchini, olive, and tomato polenta fingers

This recipe is also nut-free and gluten-free.

2 cups water
2 cups gluten-free chicken stock
1 cup polenta
1 large zucchini (5 oz), coarsely grated
½ cup (3 oz) coarsely chopped pitted
   black olives
⅓ cup (1 oz) finely grated parmesan cheese
¼ cup sun-dried tomatoes in oil, drained,
   finely chopped
2 tablespoons olive oil

1 Oil deep 7-inch-square cake pan; line base and sides with parchment.
2 Bring water and stock to the boil in large saucepan; gradually stir in polenta. Reduce heat; simmer, stirring, about 10 minutes, or until polenta thickens. Stir in zucchini, olives, cheese, and tomato. Spread polenta mixture into pan; cover, refrigerate about 1 hour or until polenta is firm.
3 Invert polenta onto board; cut in half. Cut each half into six slices.
4 Heat oil in large frying pan over medium heat; cook polenta until browned both sides.

Wrap cooled polenta fingers in parchment and place in lunchbox.

prep + cook time 25 minutes (+ refrigeration) makes 12 nutritional count per finger
105 calories; 4.5 g total fat (1 g saturated fat); 12.7 g carbohydrate; 1.1 g fiber; 2.9 g protein

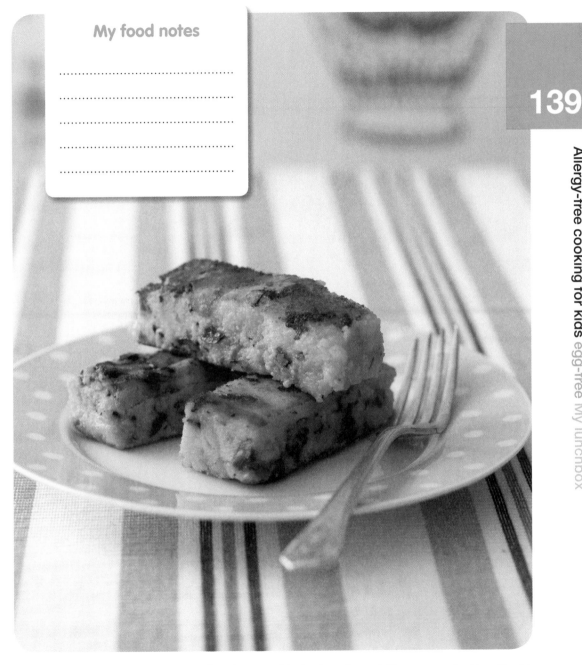

My food notes

....
....
....
....
....

Did you know? Olives are green at first then turn black when ripened. They are soaked in water or brine to remove their natural bitterness. Black olives are less bitter than the unripened green ones.

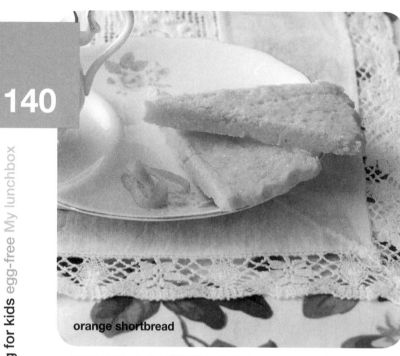

orange shortbread

prep + cook time
1 hour (+ cooling)
makes 24
nutritional count
per shortbread
145 calories;
8.6 g total fat
(5.6 g saturated fat);
16.3 g carbohydrate;
0.2 g fiber;
0.4 g protein

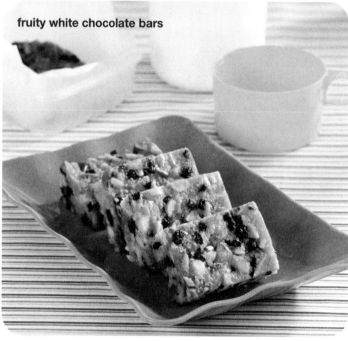

fruity white chocolate bars

prep + cook time
1 hour (+ cooling)
makes 16
nutritional count per
bar
384 calories;
22.9 g total fat
(10.3 g saturated fat);
37.1 g carbohydrate;
4.5 g fiber;
5.6 g protein

orange shortbread

This recipe is also nut-free and gluten-free.

2¼ sticks butter, softened
3 teaspoons finely grated orange rind
½ cup superfine sugar
1¾ cups gluten-free all-purpose flour
⅓ cup rice flour
1 tablespoon white sugar

1 Preheat oven to 300°F/275°F convection. Grease two baking sheets.
2 Beat butter, rind, and sugar in small bowl with electric mixer until light and fluffy. Transfer mixture to large bowl; stir in sifted flours in two batches. Knead dough lightly on floured surface until smooth.
3 Divide dough in half; shape each, on separate trays, into 8-inch rounds. Score each round into twelve wedges; prick with fork. Pinch edges of rounds with fingers; sprinkle with white sugar.
4 Bake shortbread about 40 minutes. Stand 5 minutes; using a sharp knife, cut shortbread into wedges. Cool on pans.

fruity white chocolate bars

⅔ cup (3 oz) slivered almonds
1¼ cups (7 oz) Brazil nuts, coarsely chopped
1½ cups desiccated (dried) coconut
1 cup (5 oz) coarsely chopped dried apricots
1 cup (5 oz) dried currants
¼ cup all-purpose flour
9 oz white chocolate, chopped and melted
½ cup apricot jam
½ cup honey

1 Preheat oven to 325°F/300°F convection. Grease 7 x 11-inch rectangular cake pan; line base and two long sides with parchment, extending paper 2 inches over sides.
2 Combine nuts, coconut, fruit, and flour in large bowl. Stir in combined hot melted chocolate, sieved jam, and honey. Spread evenly into prepared pan.
3 Bake about 45 minutes. Cool in pan before cutting into pieces.

chicken and vegetable soup

This recipe is also nut-free and dairy-free.

1 cup water

5 cups chicken stock

2 stalks celery (7 oz), trimmed,
thinly sliced

2 medium carrots (8 oz), diced into
⅓-inch pieces

1 large potato (11 oz), diced into
⅓-inch pieces

5 oz snow peas, trimmed,
coarsely chopped

3 scallions, thinly sliced

11 oz can corn kernels, drained

3 cups coarsely shredded
cooked chicken meat

1 Place water and stock in large saucepan; bring to a boil. Add celery, carrot, and potato; return to a boil. Reduce heat; simmer, covered, about 10 minutes, or until vegetables are just tender.

2 Add snow peas, scallions, and corn to soup; cook, covered, 2 minutes. Add chicken; stir until heated through.

prep + cook time 25 minutes (+ refrigeration) serves 4 nutritional count per serving
303 calories, 8.2 g total fat (2.4 g saturated fat); 26.9 g carbohydrate; 6.3 g fiber; 27.2 g protein

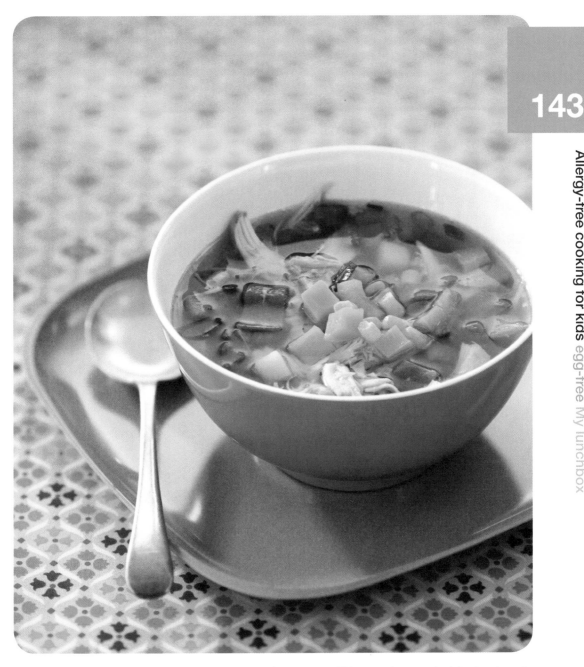

Handy hint Pack the soup in a small thermos to keep warm. This soup is a great winter lunch and will have school friends wishing they could have some too. Egg-free noodles may also be added.

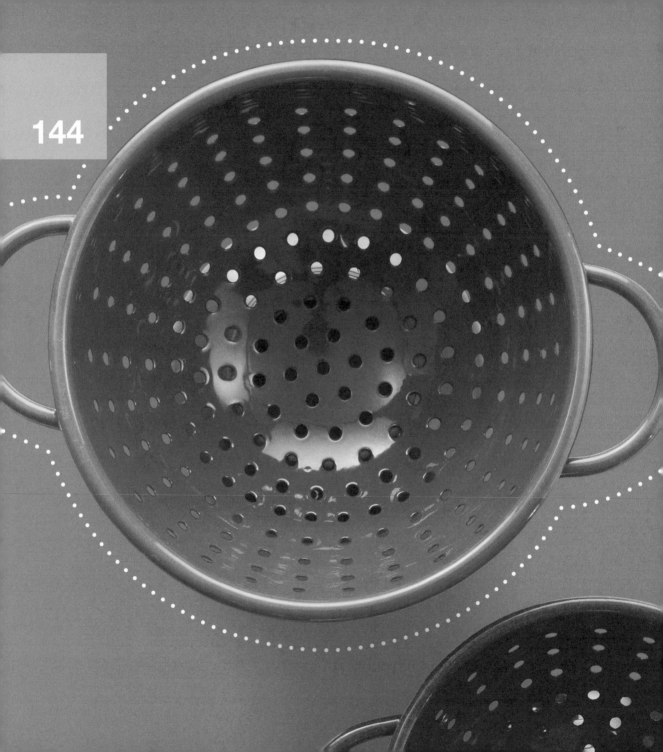

My favorite recipes

....
....
....
....
....
....
....
....

After-school snacks Need some energy to get that homework done? Then try a sweet potato biscuit or toasted banana bread.

kumara dampers

This recipe is also nut-free and gluten-free.

1⅔ cups gluten-free self-rising flour
1 teaspoon superfine sugar
¼ teaspoon salt
1½ tablespoons butter
½ cup cold mashed sieved
   cooked sweet potato
½ cup buttermilk
2 tablespoons water, approximately
2 teaspoons milk, approximately
2 teaspoons gluten-free self-rising
   flour, extra

1 Preheat oven to 425°F/400°F convection. Oil baking sheet.
2 Sift dry ingredients into large bowl; rub in the butter. Add potato, buttermilk, and enough of the water to mix to a soft, sticky dough. Knead dough lightly on floured surface until smooth.
3 Divide dough into four equal portions. Roll each portion into rounds, place on pan. Cut cross through top of dough, about ¼-inch deep. Brush tops with milk, then dust with extra sifted flour.
4 Bake biscuits about 35 minutes.

prep + cook time 50 minutes makes 4 nutritional count per damper 130 calories; 5.2 g total fat (3.2 g saturated fat); 56.5 g carbohydrate; 1.5 g fiber; 2.8 g protein

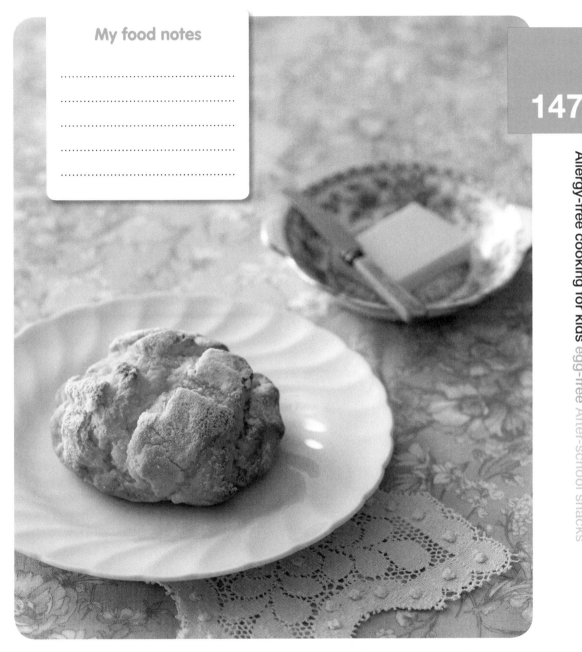

My food notes

....
....
....
....
....

Handy hint You need to cook 8 oz sweet potatoes for this recipe. Sweet potatoes are high in beta-carotene, which is converted to vitamin A, and plays an important role in vision, bone development, and the body's immunity.

Allergy-free cooking for kids egg-free After-school snacks

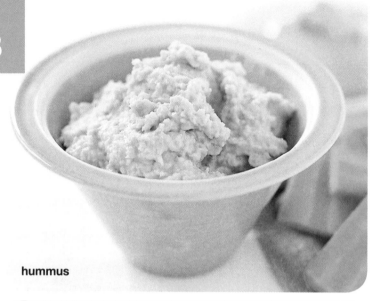

hummus

prep time
10 minutes
serves 4
nutritional count
per serving
429 calories;
36.7 g total fat
(5.1 g saturated fat);
14.4 g carbohydrate;
6.3 g fiber;
8.5 g protein

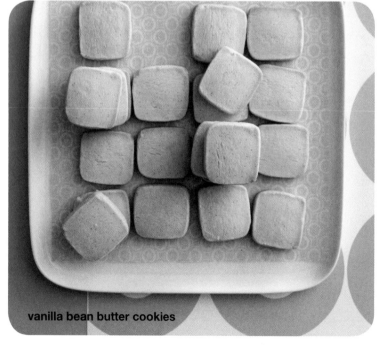

vanilla bean butter cookies

prep + cook time
30 minutes
(+ refrigeration)
makes 22
nutritional count
per biscuit
68 calories;
4.5 g total fat
(2.9 g saturated fat);
6.4 g carbohydrate;
0.1 g fiber;
0.5 g protein

hummus

This recipe is also gluten-free and dairy-free.

2 10½ oz cans chickpeas, rinsed, drained
2 tablespoons tahini (sesame seed paste)
⅓ cup lemon juice
2 cloves garlic, quartered
¼ cup water
½ cup olive oil

1 Blend or process chickpeas with tahini, juice, garlic, and water until almost smooth.
2 With motor operating, gradually add oil in a thin, steady stream until mixture forms a smooth paste.

Serve hummus with your choice of crudités (thin slices of fresh vegetables).

vanilla bean butter cookies

This recipe is also nut-free.

1 stick butter, softened
½ cup confectioners' sugar
1 vanilla bean
1¼ cups all-purpose flour

1 Place butter and sifted confectioners' sugar in small bowl. Split vanilla bean; scrape seeds into bowl. Beat with electric mixer until light and fluffy; stir in sifted flour, in two batches.
2 Knead dough on floured surface until smooth. Shape dough into 10-inch rectangular log. Enclose log in plastic wrap; refrigerate about 30 minutes or until firm.
3 Preheat oven to 350°F/325°F convection. Grease baking sheets; line with parchment.
4 Cut log into ⅓-inch slices; place slices about ½-inch apart on pans. Bake about 12 minutes. Cool on pan.

banana bread

This recipe is also gluten-free and dairy-free.

2 tablespoons desiccated (dried) coconut
1½ cups mashed overripe banana
    (see handy hint, page 151)
1¼ cups firmly packed brown sugar
½ cup vegetable oil
2 teaspoons gluten-free baking powder
1 teaspoon pie spice
2½ cups desiccated (dried) coconut, extra
1¾ cups linseed, sunflower, and ground
    almonds (LSA)

1 Preheat oven to 350°F/325°F convection. Grease 4½ x 8½-inch loaf pan; coat base and sides with desiccated coconut. Shake out excess coconut.

2 Combine banana, sugar, oil, baking powder, and pie spice in large bowl; stir in extra coconut and LSA. Spread mixture into pan; smooth surface.

3 Bake bread about 55 minutes. Stand in pan 10 minutes; invert onto parchment-covered wire rack to cool. Good eaten either fresh or toasted the next day.

prep + cook time 1 hour 10 minutes (+ cooling) makes 10 slices nutritional count per slice
507 calories; 34.3 g total fat (16.2 g saturated fat); 41.4 g carbohydrate; 5 g fiber; 7.4 g protein

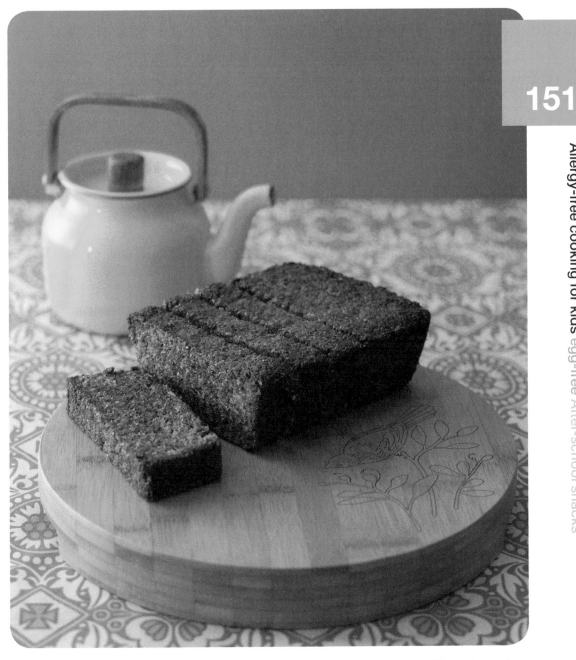

Handy hints You need 3 large overripe bananas for this recipe. LSA, a mixture of linseeds, sunflower seeds, and ground almonds, is available in health-food shops or the health-food aisle of supermarkets.

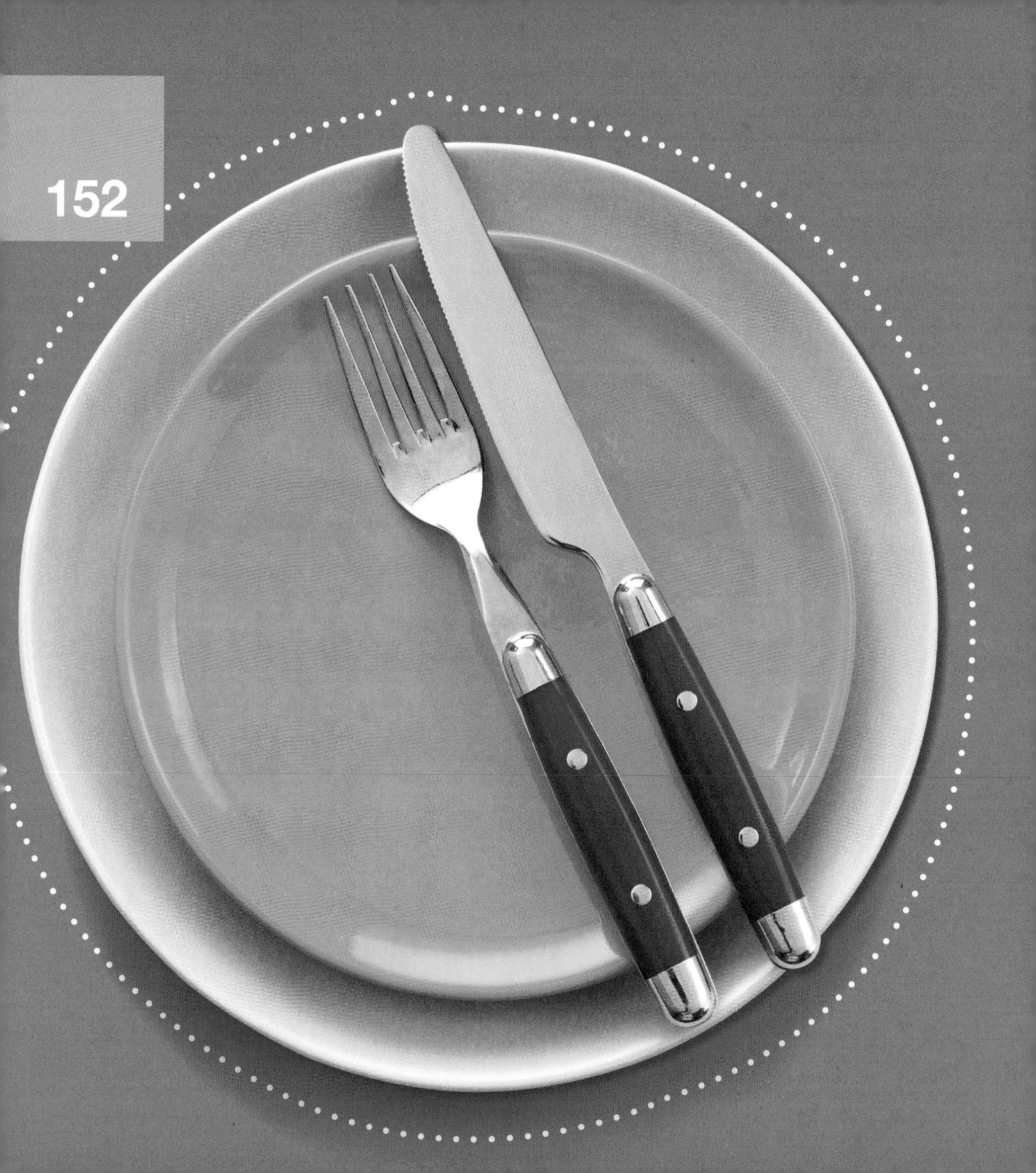

My favorite recipes

....

....

....

....

....

....

....

....

....

Dinner for everyone Keep the family and, more importantly, the cook happy with these delicious dinners for everyone.

minty lamb cutlets with mixed veggie smash

This recipe is also nut-free and dairy-free.

1 tablespoon finely chopped fresh mint
⅓ cup mint jelly
1 teaspoon finely grated lemon rind
2 teaspoons olive oil
8 french-trimmed lamb cutlets (14 oz)
mixed veggie smash
1⅓ lbs baby new potatoes, halved
2 large carrots (13 oz), cut into ½-inch pieces
1 cup (4 oz) frozen peas
1 tablespoon olive oil
1 tablespoon lemon juice
2 tablespoons finely chopped fresh mint

1 Make mixed veggie smash.

2 Combine mint and jelly in small bowl.

3 Rub combined rind and oil over lamb; cook lamb on heated oiled grill pan (or grill or barbecue) until cooked as you like.

4 Serve lamb with veggie smash and mint mixture.

mixed veggie smash Boil, steam, or microwave potato, carrot, and peas, separately, until tender; drain. Crush potato and peas roughly in large bowl; stir in carrot and remaining ingredients.

prep + cook time 40 minutes serves 4 nutritional count per serving 376 calories; 15.8 g total fat (4.9 g saturated fat); 38.4 g carbohydrate; 7.3 g fiber; 16.3 g protein

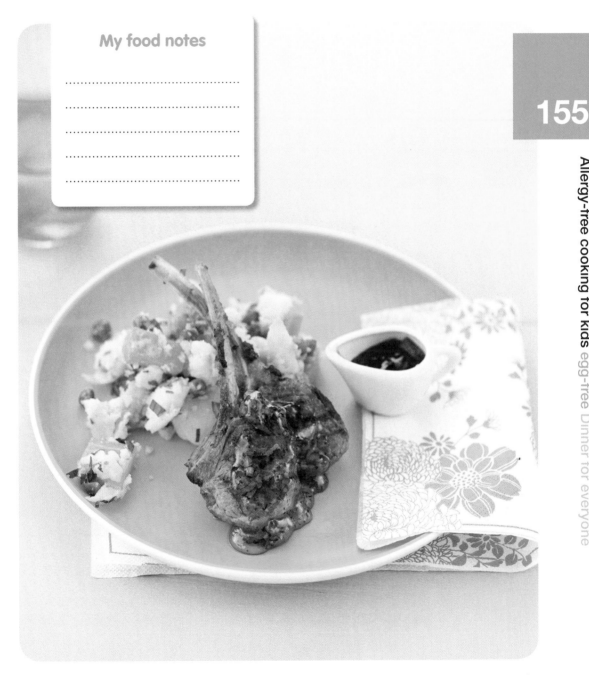

Did you know? "French-trimmed" is a butcher's term referring to a cutting method where excess sinew, gristle, and fat from the bone end of cutlets, racks, or shanks are removed and the bones are cleaned.

Allergy-free cooking for kids egg-free Dinner for everyone

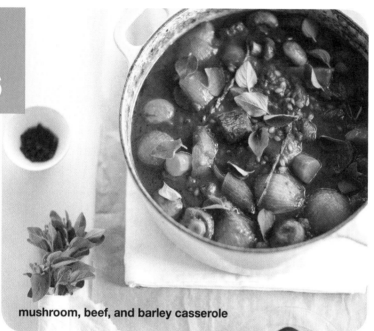

mushroom, beef, and barley casserole

prep + cook time
3 hours 15 minutes
serves 4
nutritional count
per serving
682 calories;
22.4 g total fat
(6.3 g saturated fat);
43 g carbohydrate;
11.5 g fiber;
60.5 g protein

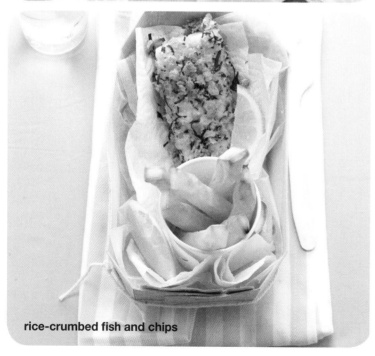

rice-crumbed fish and chips

prep + cook time
1 hour serves 4
nutritional count
per serving
386 calories;
5.6 g total fat
(1.8 g saturated fat);
43.2 g carbohydrate;
4.8 g fiber;
37.4 g protein

mushroom, beef, and barley casserole

This is also nut-free and dairy free.

2 tablespoons olive oil
2 lbs beef chuck steak, cut into 1-inch cubes
large pearl onions (11 oz), halved
2 medium carrots (8 oz), coarsely chopped
2 cups beef stock
2 14 oz cans diced tomatoes
2 sprigs fresh rosemary
7 black peppercorns
7 oz button mushrooms
½ cup pearl barley
2 tablespoons fresh oregano leaves

1 Preheat oven to 350°F/325°F convection.
2 Heat half the oil in large flameproof casserole dish over medium-high heat; cook beef, in batches, until browned.
3 Heat remaining oil in same dish; cook onion and carrot, stirring, until vegetables soften. Return beef to dish with stock, undrained tomatoes, rosemary, and peppercorns; bring to the boil. Cover, transfer to oven; cook, 2 hours, stirring occasionally.
4 Stir in mushrooms and barley, return to oven; cook, uncovered, 45 minutes or until barley is tender. Serve garnished with oregano.

rice-crumbed fish and chips

This recipe is also nut-free, gluten-free and dairy-free.

4 medium potatoes (1¾ lbs)
1⅓ cup rice flakes
2 tablespoons finely chopped fresh
    flat-leaf parsley
1 tablespoon finely grated lemon rind
1⅓ lbs firm white fish filets, halved
    lengthwise
cooking oil spray

1 Preheat oven to 425°F/400°F convection.
2 Cut potato into ⅓-inch slices; cut slices into ⅓-inch fries. Place fries on parchment-lined baking sheet; bake about 35 minutes or until browned lightly.
3 Meanwhile, coarsely crush rice flakes in small bowl; mix in parsley and rind. Press crumb mixture onto both sides of fish; spray fish on each side with cooking oil spray.
4 Place fish on pan; cook in oven for final 10 minutes of potato-cooking time.
5 Divide fish and chips between four serving plates.

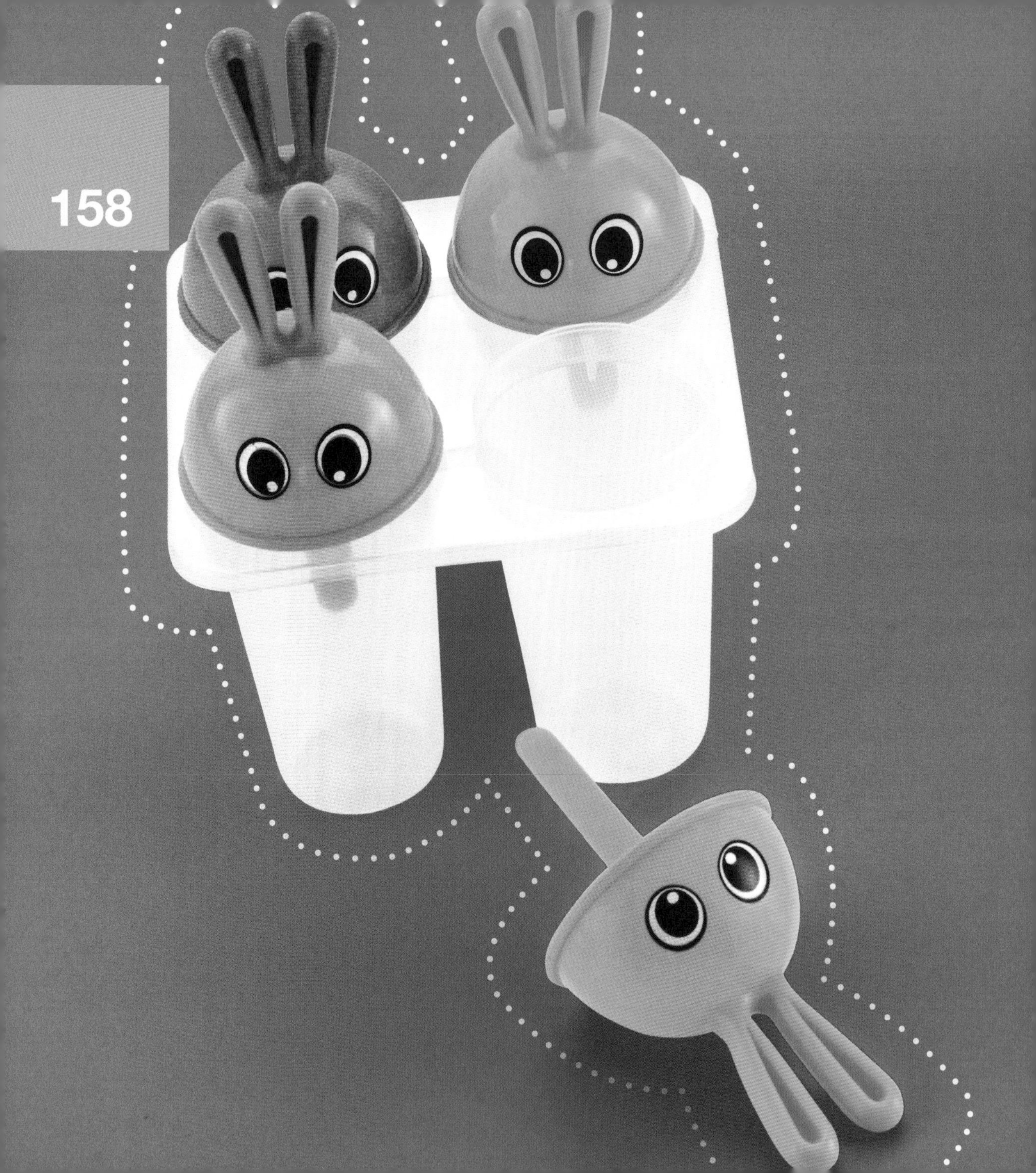

My favorite recipes

....

....

....

....

....

....

....

....

Seriously sweet Puddings, crumbles, turnovers—so many scrumptious recipes to choose from without an egg to be seen.

apple and pear crumble

This recipe is also gluten-free.

3 medium apples (1 lb)
3 medium pears (1½ lbs)
¼ cup superfine sugar
¼ cup water
crumble topping
½ cup (2 oz) ground almonds
⅓ cup rice flour
⅓ cup firmly packed brown sugar
4 tablespoons butter, chopped
1 teaspoon ground cinnamon

1 Preheat oven to 350°F/325°F convection. Grease deep 1½-quart ovenproof dish.
2 Peel, core, and quarter apples and pears; thickly slice fruit. Combine fruit, sugar, and the water in large saucepan; cook, covered, about 10 minutes, or until fruit is just tender. Drain; discard liquid.
3 Meanwhile, make crumble topping.
4 Place apple mixture in dish; sprinkle the topping over. Bake crumble about 25 minutes.

crumble topping Blend or process ingredients until combined.

variations

granola crumble Prepare half the amount of basic crumble mixture; stir in 1 cup toasted granola. (Note: this is not a gluten-free crumble.)

coconut crumble Prepare half the amount of basic crumble mixture; stir in ½ cup shredded coconut.

prep + cook time 45 minutes serves 4 nutritional count per serving 522 calories; 21 g total fat (8.7 g saturated fat); 75.2 g carbohydrate; 5.8 g fiber; 4.8 g protein

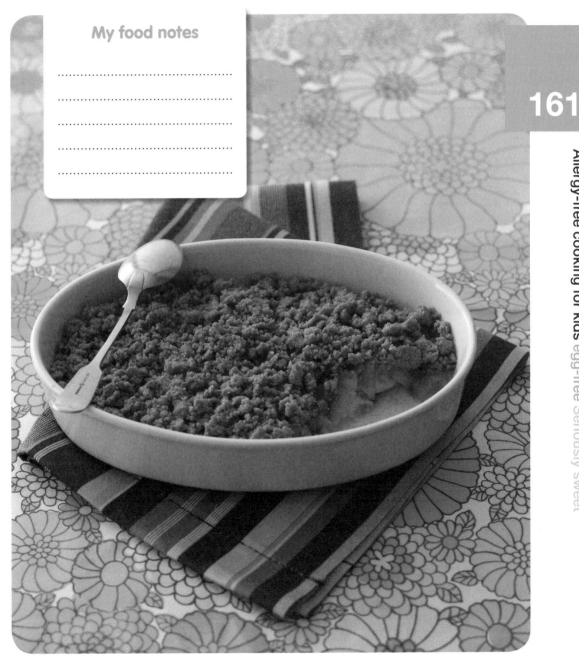

My food notes

....
....
....
....
....

Handy hint Golden Delicious apples are a crisp almost citrus-colored apple with an excellent flavor and are a good choice for this dish. The popular Granny Smith apple is also a good choice.

Allergy-free cooking for kids egg-free Seriously sweet

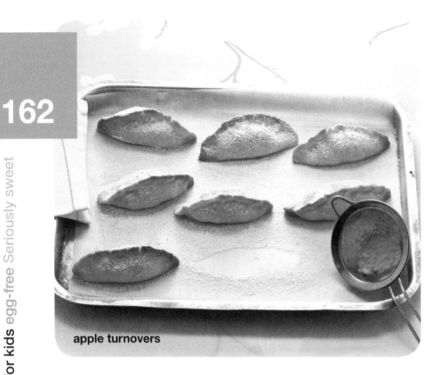

apple turnovers

prep + cook time
40 minutes
makes 18
nutritional count
per turnover
151 calories;
7.2 g total fat
(4.6 g saturated fat);
19.6 g carbohydrate;
0.7 g fiber;
1.7 g protein

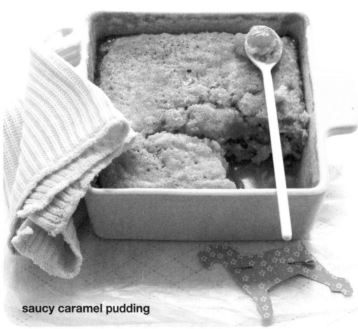

saucy caramel pudding

prep + cook time
1 hour 10 minutes
serves 4
nutritional count
per serving
289 calories;
11.7 g total fat
(7.6 g saturated fat);
67.1 g carbohydrate;
0.5 g fiber;
1.7 g protein

apple turnovers

This recipe is also nut-free and gluten-free.

2 medium apples (11 oz), peeled,
  finely chopped
1 teaspoon superfine sugar
2 tablespoons water
1 teaspoon confectioners' sugar
gluten-free pastry
1¼ cups rice flour
¼ cup (100% corn) cornstarch
¼ cup soy flour
⅓ cup superfine sugar
1¼ sticks cold butter, coarsely chopped
2 tablespoons cold water, approximately

1 Preheat oven to 400°F/375°F convection. Grease and line baking sheet with parchment.
2 Make gluten-free pastry.
3 Combine apple, sugar, and the water in saucepan; bring to the boil. Reduce heat; simmer, covered, 5 minutes, or until apple is tender. Cool.
4 Roll pastry between sheets of parchment until ¼-inch thick; cut out eighteen 3-inch rounds. Drop heaping teaspoons of apple mixture into center of each round; fold to enclose filling, pinching edges.
5 Place turnovers on sheet. Bake, in oven, about 15 minutes; cool on sheet. Serve dusted with sifted confectioners' sugar.
gluten-free pastry Process flours, sugar, and butter until crumbly. Add enough of the water to make a dough. Knead gently on floured surface until smooth.

saucy caramel pudding

This recipe is also nut-free and gluten-free.

1 cup gluten-free self-rising flour
⅓ cup firmly packed brown sugar
1½ tablespoons butter, melted
½ cup milk
caramel sauce
1⅓ cups water
⅓ cup firmly packed brown sugar
2 tablespoons butter

1 Preheat oven to 350°F/325°F convection. Grease deep 1-quart ovenproof dish.
2 Combine sifted flour, sugar, butter, and milk in medium bowl. Pour batter into dish.
3 Make caramel sauce.
4 Pour sauce slowly and evenly over back of a spoon over batter in dish. Bake pudding about 50 minutes. Stand 10 minutes before serving.
caramel sauce Combine ingredients in small saucepan; stir over medium heat, without boiling, until smooth.

self-saucing jaffa pudding

This recipe is also nut-free and gluten-free.

4½ tablespoons butter
½ cup milk
½ teaspoon vanilla extract
¾ cup superfine sugar
½ cup rice flour
⅓ cup soy flour
⅓ cup gluten-free self-rising flour
1 teaspoon gluten-free baking powder
2 tablespoons cocoa powder
2 teaspoons finely grated orange rind
½ cup firmly packed brown sugar
2 cups boiling water

1 Preheat oven to 350°F/325°F convection. Grease 1½-quart ovenproof dish.
2 Melt butter with milk and extract in medium saucepan over low heat. Remove from heat; whisk in sugar, then sifted flours, baking powder, half the cocoa, and rind. Spread mixture into dish.
3 Sift brown sugar and the remaining cocoa over batter; gently pour the boiling water over batter.
4 Bake pudding about 40 minutes. Stand 5 minutes before serving.

prep + cook time 1 hour serves 6 nutritional count per serving 375 calories; 11 g total fat (6.4 g saturated fat); 68.1 g carbohydrate; 1.3 g fiber; 4.8 g protein

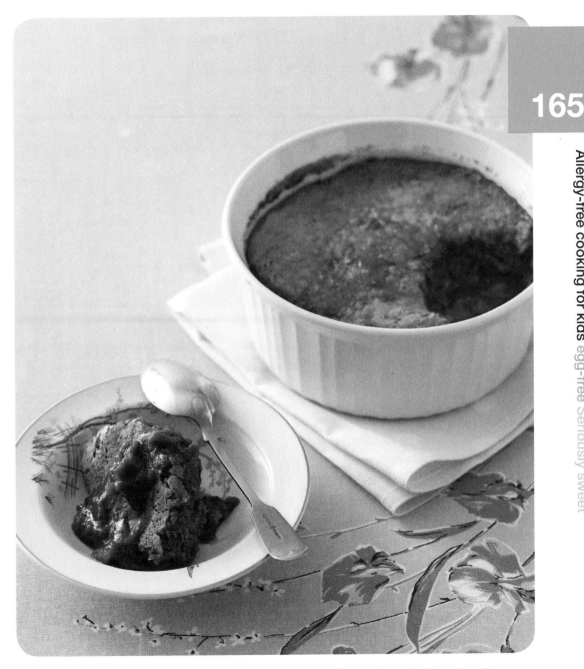

Did you know? Jaffa is sometimes used to describe a small round sweet with a chocolate-orange flavor. It is also a type of sweet orange grown in Israel; it takes its name from the city of Jaffa.

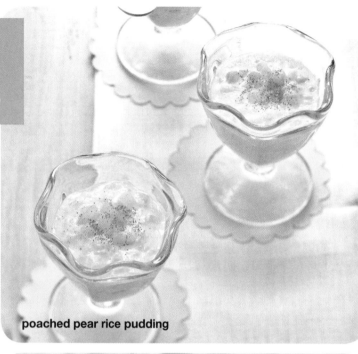

poached pear rice pudding

prep + cook time
1¼ hour serves 6
nutritional count
per serving
204 calories;
6.6 g total fat
(4.3 g saturated fat);
29 g carbohydrate;
0.8 g fiber;
6.5 g protein

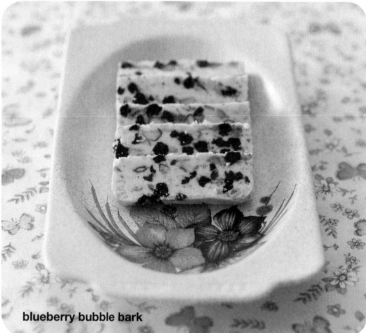

blueberry bubble bark

prep + cook time
15 minutes
(+ refrigeration)
makes 16
nutritional count
per slice
97 calories;
6.5 g total fat
(3.9 g saturated fat);
7.9 g carbohydrate;
0.7 g fiber;
1.5 g protein

poached pear rice pudding

This recipe is also nut-free and gluten-free.

1 quart milk
¼ cup superfine sugar
⅓ cup white medium-grain rice, washed, drained
2 cups water
1 small pear (6 oz), peeled, halved
1 cinnamon stick

1 Combine milk and sugar in medium saucepan; bring to the boil, stirring occasionally. Gradually stir in rice; simmer, uncovered, stirring occasionally, about 40 minutes, or until rice is tender.
2 Meanwhile, combine the water, pear, and cinnamon stick in small saucepan; bring to the boil. Simmer, uncovered, about 20 minutes, or until pear is tender. Remove pear from liquid, finely chop; reserve 2 teaspoons, stir remaining pear into pudding. Top with reserved pear. Serve warm.

blueberry bubble bark

This recipe is also gluten-free.

6 oz white chopped chocolate, melted
¾ cup puffed rice
½ cup desiccated (dried) coconut
½ cup (3 oz) dried blueberries
¼ cup (1 oz) unsalted pistachios, coarsely chopped

1 Grease 3 x 10-inch tart pan; line base and two long sides with parchment, extending paper 2 inches above sides.
2 Combine ingredients in medium bowl.
3 Spoon mixture evenly into pan; refrigerate until set. Remove bark slice from pan; cut into slices.

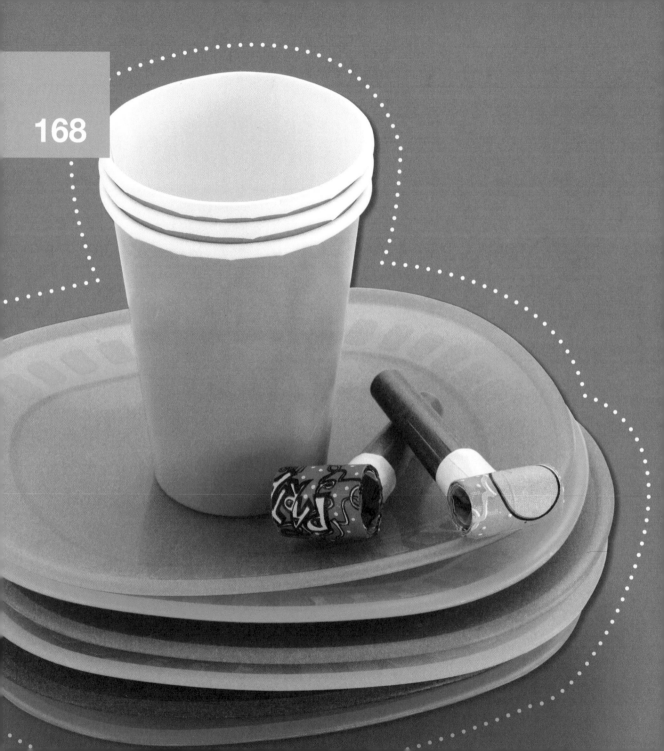

My favorite recipes

....
....
....
....
....
....
....
....
....

Party time No one will go hungry at this party—there's plenty to go around so that even hungry adults will get a bite to eat.

mini beef meatballs

This recipe is also nut-free.

2 lbs ground beef
1 cup stale breadcrumbs
½ cup (1½ oz) coarsely grated
   parmesan cheese
2 cloves garlic, crushed
2 scallions, thinly sliced
1 tablespoon Worcestershire sauce
2 tablespoons barbecue sauce
2 tablespoons olive oil

1 Combine beef, breadcrumbs, cheese, garlic, onion, and sauces in large bowl; shape level tablespoons of mixture into balls.
2 Heat oil in large frying pan over medium heat; cook meatballs, in batches, until cooked through. Drain on paper towels.
3 Serve meatballs with tomato sauce.

The meatballs can be cooked one day ahead and kept, covered, in the refrigerator. Reheat meatballs, in single layer, on baking sheets, covered loosely with foil, in 350°F/325°F convection oven for about 10 minutes. Freeze uncooked meatballs between layers of freezer wrap for 3 months; thaw in the refrigerator for 12 hours or overnight before cooking as per recipe.

prep + cook time 45 minutes makes 55 nutritional count per meatball 51 calories; 2 g total fat (0.3 g saturated fat); 5.8 g carbohydrate; 1.6 g fiber; 2.2 g protein

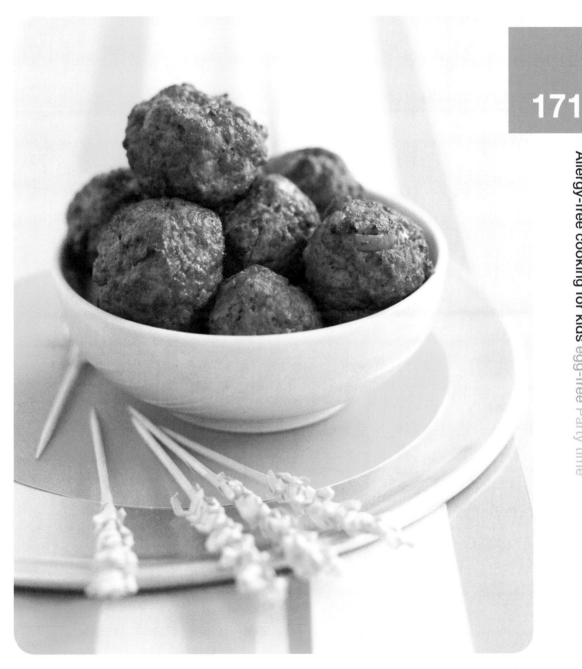

Handy hint Simmer the meatballs in your favorite tomato-based sauce and serve with spaghetti for a delicious helping of spaghetti and meatballs. Garnish with parmesan cheese before serving.

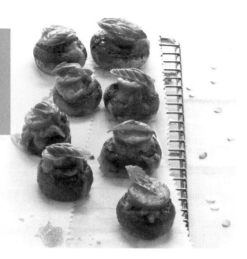

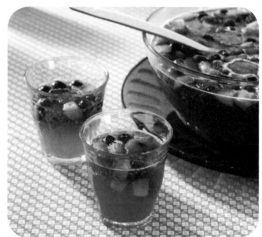

mushroom cups

24 button mushrooms (10½ oz)
½ cup bottled basil pesto
12 cherry tomatoes, halved
½ cup (2 oz) coarsely grated
  cheddar cheese
24 small basil leaves

1 Remove stems from mushrooms; place, top-side down, on foiled-lined pan. Divide pesto between mushroom cups; top each with a tomato half, cut-side up, sprinkle cheese over them.
2 Preheat broiler.
3 Broil mushrooms about 5 minutes or until cheese melts. Serve each topped with a basil leaf.

prep + cook time 25 minutes makes 24
nutritional count per mushroom cup
35 calories; 3 g total fat (1 g saturated fat);
0.2 g carbohydrate; 0.5 g fiber; 1.6 g protein

berry punch

This recipe is also dairy-free.

8 oz strawberries
1 quart tropical fruit punch juice
1 quart chilled dry ginger ale
1 cup (4 oz) blueberries
1 cup (4 oz) raspberries
2 teaspoons grenadine-flavored syrup

1 Finely chop half the strawberries. Divide into 12-hole (1 tablespoon) ice-cube tray. Pour 1 cup of the juice into the holes; freeze overnight.
2 Coarsely chop remaining strawberries; combine in large punch bowl or pitcher with remaining juice, ginger ale, strawberry ice cubes, blueberries, raspberries, and grenadine.

prep time 15 minutes (+ freezing)
makes 2 liters nutritional count per 1 cup
113 calories; 0.4 g total fat (0 g saturated fat);
38 g carbohydrate; 1.8 g fiber; 1 g protein

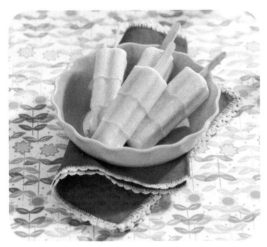

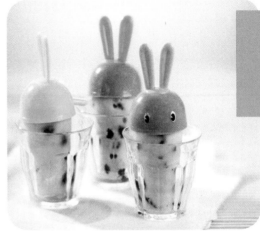

honey and banana ice pops

1 large banana (8 oz), coarsely chopped
⅔ cup vanilla yogurt
1 tablespoon honey

1 Blend or process ingredients until smooth and creamy.
2 Pour into four ⅓-cup popsicle molds. Freeze overnight until firm.

preparation time 5 minutes (+ freezing)
makes 4 nutritional count per ice-block
104 calories; 1.7 g total fat (1.1 g saturated fat); 18.4 g carbohydrate; 0.8 g fiber; 3.1 g protein

fruity yogurt ice pops

1½ cups vanilla yogurt
1 cup (5 oz) frozen mixed berries
1 tablespoon honey

1 Combine ingredients in medium bowl.
2 Spoon into six ¼-cup popsicle molds. Press lids on firmly; freeze overnight until firm.

preparation time 5 minutes (+ freezing)
makes 6 nutritional count per ice-block
91 calories; 2.4 g total fat (1.5 g saturated fat); 12.5 g carbohydrate; 1 g fiber; 3.8 g protein

chocolate marshmallow squares

2 tablespoons powdered gelatin
½ cup water
2 cups superfine sugar
1 cup water, extra
½ teaspoon lemon extract
¼ teaspoon yellow food coloring
10½ oz white chocolate, finely grated

1 Grease 8 x 12-inch cake pan; line base and sides with plastic wrap.

2 Sprinkle gelatin over the water in small bowl.

3 Combine sugar and the extra water in large saucepan. Stir over heat, without boiling, until sugar dissolves; bring to the boil. Add gelatin mixture; boil steadily, uncovered, about 10 minutes or until mixture is thick but not changed in color.

4 Pour sugar mixture into large heatproof bowl of electric mixer; add extract and coloring. Beat on high speed about 5 minutes or until mixture is very thick and holds its shape.

5 Spread marshmallow mixture into pan. Stand at room temperature about 2 hours, or until firm.

6 Using wet knife, cut marshmallow into ¾-inch squares; roll squares in chocolate.

prep + cook time 30 minutes (+ refrigeration and standing) makes 48 nutritional count per square 73 calories; 2.1 g total fat (1.3 g saturated fat); 12.6 g carbohydrate; 0 g fiber; 0.9 g protein

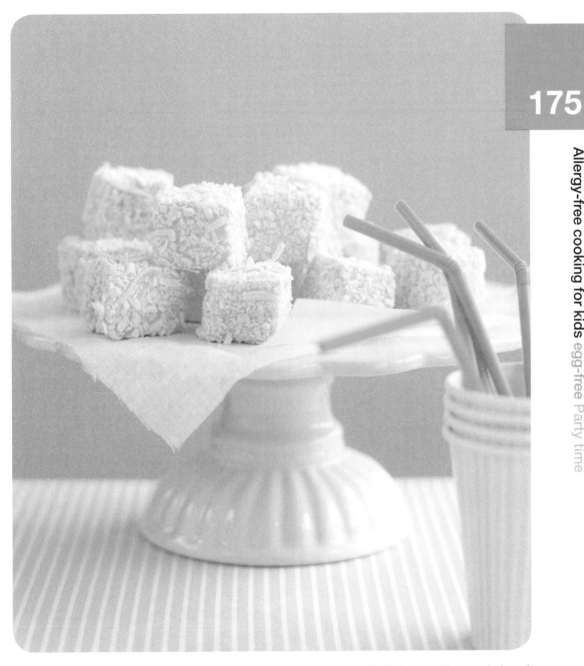

Handy hint Add some extra color to the marshmallow by tinting half of it lightly with your choice of food coloring—the range is limitless and can be added to suit the color theme of your party.

glossary

arrowroot a starch made from a rhizome of a Central American plant; used mostly as a thickener.

baking powder a rising agent; consists of two parts cream of tartar to one part baking soda. Gluten-free baking powder is made without cereals.

baking soda a rising agent; also called bicarbonate soda.

cheese
cream commonly called Philadelphia or Philly, a soft cow's milk cheese.
mascarpone a fresh cultured-cream product made like yogurt. Whiteish to creamy yellow with a buttery-rich texture.
pizza a blend of grated mozzarella, cheddar, and parmesan cheeses.

chocolate
bittersweet (70% cocoa solids) made of a high percentage of cocoa liquor and cocoa butter, and little added sugar. We use bittersweet chocolate unless stated otherwise.
white contains no cocoa solids, deriving its sweetness from cocoa butter. Very sensitive to heat.

cilantro, fresh also known as pak chee, coriander, or Chinese parsley; bright-green-leafed herb with a pungent flavor.

cornflakes, gluten-free available from health-food stores and some supermarkets.

cornstarch also known as cornflour; used as a thickening agent. Available as 100% corn (maize) and wheaten cornstarch.

cream of tartar acid ingredient in baking powder; used in confectionery mixtures to help prevent sugar from crystallizing.

cream we use heavy cream (also known as pure cream).

cream, sour thick, commercially-cultured sour cream with at least 35% fat content.

flaxseed meal ground flax seeds. Available from health-food stores and some supermarkets.

flour
all-purpose flour made from wheat. It is also available as gluten-free from health-food shops and most supermarkets.
bread mix, gluten-free a commercial gluten-free bread mix available from most supermarkets and health-food stores.
buckwheat not a true cereal, but flour is made from its seeds. Available from health-food stores.
chickpea also called besan or gram; made from ground chickpeas so is gluten-free and high in protein.
potato made from cooked potatoes that have been dried and ground.
rice very fine, almost powdery, gluten-free flour; made from ground white rice.
self-rising all-purpose flour mixed with baking powder in the proportion of 1 cup flour to 2 teaspoons baking powder. Gluten-free is also available from most supermarkets and health-food stores.
soy made from ground soy beans.

garam masala a blend of cardamom, cinnamon, cloves, cilantro, fennel, and cumin, roasted and ground together.

gelatin we use powdered gelatin. It is also available in sheet form (leaf gelatin).

glacé fruit (cherries, pineapple, etc.) when buying glacé fruit check the ingredients label for "glucose made from wheat"; glacé fruit is available without glucose, making it gluten-free and wheat-free.

golden syrup a by-product of sugarcane.

linseed, sunflower, and almond meal (LSA) available from health-food stores and some supermarkets.

mandarin also called tangerine. Mandarin juice is available in the refrigerated section in most supermarkets.

maple syrup, pure distilled from the sap of maple trees. Maple-flavored syrup or pancake syrup is not an adequate substitute for the real thing.

noodles, rice vermicelli also called sen mee, mei fun, or bee hoon; used in spring rolls and salads. Before using, soak dried noodles in hot water until softened, boil briefly then rinse with hot water.

oil

hazelnut a mono-unsaturated oil, pressed from crushed hazelnuts.

macadamia oil is extracted from ground macadamias. Available in some larger supermarkets and delicatessens.

onions

red also called Spanish, red Spanish, or Bermuda onion; a sweet-flavored, large, purple-red onion.

scallion an immature onion picked before the bulb has formed, having a long, bright-green edible stalk.

pancetta an Italian unsmoked bacon; pork belly cured in salt and spices then rolled into a sausage shape and dried for several weeks.

polenta also called cornmeal; a flour-like cereal made of corn (maize). Also the dish made from it.

poppy seeds small, dried, bluish-gray seeds; crunchy and nutty. Available whole or ground from most supermarkets.

rice flakes, gluten-free available from the health-food section in most supermarkets.

rice, rolled flattened rice grain rolled into flakes; looks similar to rolled oats.

sugar

brown a soft, finely granulated sugar with molasses for its color and flavor.

superfine also called caster or finely granulated table sugar.

white a coarse, granulated table sugar, also called crystal sugar.

vanilla

bean dried, long, thin pod from a tropical golden orchid; the minuscule black seeds inside the bean are used to impart a luscious vanilla flavor.

extract vanilla beans are pulped into a mixture with alcohol and water. Only a couple of drops are needed.

zucchini also known as courgette; small members of the squash family.

conversion chart

measures

All cup and spoon measurements are level. The most accurate way to measure dry ingredients is to use a spoon to fill the measuring cup, without packing or scooping with the cup, and leveling off the top with a straight edge.

When measuring liquids, use a clear glass or plastic liquid measuring cup with markings on the side.

Unless otherwise indicated, always work with room-temperature ingredients. Cold liquids added to butter can cause any batters and icings to break. We use large eggs averaging 2 ounces each.

dry measures

IMPERIAL	METRIC
½ oz	15 g
1 oz	30 g
2 oz	60 g
3 oz	90 g
4 oz (¼ lb)	125 g
5 oz	155 g
6 oz	185 g
7 oz	220 g
8 oz (½ lb)	250 g
9 oz	280 g
10 oz	315 g
11 oz	345 g
12 oz (¾ lb)	375 g
13 oz	410 g
14 oz	440 g
15 oz	470 g
16 oz (1 lb)	500 g
24 oz (1½ lb)	750 g
32 oz (2 lb)	1 kg

liquid measures

IMPERIAL	METRIC
1 fluid oz	30 ml
2 fluid oz	60 ml
3 fluid oz	100 ml
4 fluid oz	125 ml
5 fluid oz (¼ pint/1 gill)	150 ml
6 fluid oz	190 ml
8 fluid oz	250 ml
10 fluid oz (½ pint)	300 ml
16 fluid oz	500 ml
20 fluid oz (1 pint)	600 ml
1¾ pints	1000 ml (1 liter)

length measures

IMPERIAL	METRIC
⅛ in	3 mm
¼ in	6 mm
½ in	1 cm
¾ in	2 cm
1 in	2.5 cm
2 in	5 cm
2½ in	6 cm
3 in	8 cm
4 in	10 cm
5 in	13 cm
6 in	15 cm
7 in	18 cm
8 in	20 cm
9 in	23 cm
10 in	25 cm
11 in	28 cm
12 in (1 ft)	30 cm

oven temperatures

These oven temperatures are only a guide for conventional ovens. For convection ovens, check the manufacturer's manual.

	°F (FAHRENHEIT)	°C (CELSIUS)
Very slow	250	120
Slow	275–300	150
Moderately slow	325	160
Moderate	350–375	180
Moderately hot	400	200
Hot	425–450	220
Very hot	475	240

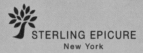

STERLING EPICURE
New York

An Imprint of Sterling Publishing
387 Park Avenue South
New York, NY 10016

ISBN 978-1-4549-1023-7

Distributed in Canada by Sterling Publishing
c/o Canadian Manda Group, 165 Dufferin Street
Toronto, Ontario, Canada M6K 3H6

For information about custom editions, special sales, and premium and corporate purchases,
please contact Sterling Special Sales at 800-805-5489 or specialsales@sterlingpublishing.com.

Manufactured in Canada

2 4 6 8 10 9 7 5 3

www.sterlingpublishing.com